Recognising LGB Sexual Identities in Health Services

The Experiences of Lesbian, Gay and Bisexual People with Health Services in North West Ireland

Maria Gibbons, Mary Manandhar, Caoimhe Gleeson and Joan Mullan

First published in December 2007 by

The Equality Authority and the Health Service Executive

© 2007 The Equality Authority and the Health Service Executive

ISBN: 978-1-905628-70-4

Design by form

Printed in Ireland by Brunswick Press

FOREWORD

This research project is unique and important in giving a voice to lesbian, gay and bisexual (LGB) clients of health services. It breaks valuable new ground as primary qualitative research into the experiences of the LGB clients of these services. It removes the invisibility that all too often hides the identity, experiences and situations of LGB clients and affords a vital and new visibility to these groups.

The research poses significant challenges to providers of health services – both at the organisational level and at the individual level. These challenges relate to the capacity of organisations and of individuals to engage with clients in a manner based on assumptions of a diversity of sexual identities rather than assumptions of a heterosexual norm. They relate to the need to create a gay- and lesbian-friendly environment within which to provide services. They relate to the ability to meet the needs of LGB clients in a manner that achieves equality and values diversity. These are challenges that can be met by building on the many instances of good practice identified by LGB clients in this research.

It will be important to develop a visible and effective response to the findings and recommendations of this research. This response will sit well with the commitment already set out by the Health Service Executive (HSE), the Department of Health and Children and the Equality Authority to developing equality competence in health service provision. This equality competence involves health service providers in:

- Putting in place equality policies.
- Providing equality and diversity training for all staff.
- Developing and implementing equality action plans.
- Gathering and analysing data on groups experiencing inequality to ensure decision-making is evidence based.
- Engaging with organisations of groups experiencing inequality to ensure decision-making is participatory.
- Conducting equality impact assessments on new plans, policies and programmes.

We are grateful to the research team of Dr Maria Gibbons, Dr Mary Manandhar and Joan Mullan for the thorough and expert nature of their work. They have valuably brought forward the voice of LGB clients of health services and charted a necessary response to the issues raised by this voice. We are also grateful to Laurence Bond who managed the project for the Equality Authority and to Caoimhe Gleeson and Dr Mary Manandhar who composed the co-ordinating team for HSE West for the project. Finally, we are grateful to the 43 lesbian, gay and bisexual people who so generously gave of their time and insights during the interviews for this research.

Niall Crowley
CEO
Equality Authority

Dr Patrick Doorley
National Director of Population Health
Health Service Executive

ACKNOWLEDGEMENTS

The Health Service Executive and the Equality Authority would like to acknowledge the contributions and work of the following people:

- Ruth Charlton, Martin Cooke, Michael McMonigle and other members of the Advisory Committee
- The project co-ordinating team
- The research team
- Laurence Bond, Anne Timoney, Ciarán Ó hUltacháin and Torben Krings of the Equality Authority Research Section
- Ursula Barry, University College Dublin
- Dr Alizon Draper, University of Westminster, London
- Dr Philip Crowley, Department of Health and Children
- Dr Sean Denyer, Population Health, HSE
- Mary Scally, Population Health, HSE
- Eileen O'Neill, Population Health, HSE
- Janet Gaynor, Health Promotion, HSE West
- Eileen Weatherall, Researcher
- Beatrice Mulrooney, Public Health, HSE West
- Joan McDonald, Public Health, HSE West
- Blaithín McKiernan, Equality Office, HSE West
- Pat Gallagher and Liz Keaney from the Primary Care Centre, Markievicz House, Sligo
- Health Service staff from Mental Health services, GUM services, GP services and the Primary Care Development Unit in Donegal, Sligo and Leitrim who participated in focus groups and provided feedback on earlier drafts.

Finally, sincerest thanks and gratitude are extended to all of the research participants who so willingly and openly gave of their time and experience. Without their generous contributions, this research would not have been possible.

CONTENTS

6. Experience of Disclosure of Sexual Identity to GP Services

7. Recognition of Partners and Parenthood

8. Mental Health

9. Sexual and Gynaecological Health

10. Suggestions for Improved Health Services for LGB Clients

11. Conclusion

TABLES

ABBREVIATIONS

AIDS	Acquired Immune Deficiency Syndrome
APA	American Psychiatric Association
CIOMS	Council for International Organisations of Medical Sciences
DOHC	Department of Health and Children
ENT	Ear, Nose and Throat
GLEN	Gay and Lesbian Equality Network
GP	General Practitioner
GUM	Genito-Urinary Medicine
HIV	Human Immunodeficiency Virus
HSE	Health Service Executive
LGB	Lesbian, Gay and Bisexual
LGBT	Lesbian, Gay, Bisexual and Transgender
NESF	National Economic and Social Forum
NHS	National Health Service (UK)
NWHB	North Western Health Board
STD	Sexually Transmitted Disease
STI	Sexually Transmitted Infection
UK	United Kingdom of Great Britain and Northern Ireland
US	United States of America

EXECUTIVE SUMMARY

This report documents the experiences of lesbian, gay and bisexual (LGB) people with the health services in the north west region. Drawing upon in-depth interviews with 43 lesbian, gay or bisexual respondents, it explores their experiences as health service users and their perspectives on the quality of care that they receive. In documenting this lived experience, it illuminates the barriers that restrict LGB people from accessing health services on an equal footing and discusses how these barriers can be addressed and how good practice can be encouraged at the level of the Health Service Executive (HSE) and of the individual service providers.

Disclosure of LGB Sexual Identity to Health Care Providers

Deciding whether to tell practitioners about their LGB sexual orientation emerged as a major concern for most research participants in their interactions with health services. Indeed, it was central to all other themes arising in the study and was found to have consequences for the ensuing health care of LGB clients. Factors that encourage LGB people to be more open about their sexual identity in health care settings were clearly identified. These included the quality of the relationship with the practitioner and whether the environment: reflected a general openness to the possibility that clients can be lesbian, gay or bisexual; fostered a sense of safety in the encounter in terms of assured confidentiality; and provided a comfortable and private space for consultations to take place. The key issue in relation to these characteristics is not that clients should be expected to disclose their sexual identity but that the conditions are supportive of them disclosing it if they think it relevant and choose to do so.

Experience of Disclosure of Sexual Identity to GP Services

Many participants have never informed any GP about their sexual orientation, some have told some GPs and not others, and some have informed every GP they have encountered. In the majority of cases where interviewees informed practitioners of their LGB sexual orientation, the GP was described by the client as responding in a positive manner. Given that all interviewees attended GPs during the study period and that the nature of primary care means that an ongoing relationship between client and practitioner is likely to develop over time, it is noteworthy that the majority of general practice personnel in the present study were never made aware of the sexual identity of their LGB clients. This study suggests that there are positive health benefits for LGB people when they disclose their sexual orientation to their GP. These include a reduction in anxiety for some LGB clients (when the response from the practitioner is a positive one) and the opportunity thus provided for practitioners to offer relevant and useful information. Those clients who do not disclose their LGB identity to primary care personnel also tend to be more cautious about other information they provide to the practitioner. These outcomes, together with the finding that many interviewees would prefer to disclose their sexual identity to service providers, suggest that practitioners generally need to be sensitive and responsive to the fact that any of their clients may be lesbian, gay or bisexual whether or not this information is actually disclosed to them during consultations.

Recognition of Partners and Parenthood

Many respondents raised concerns about the status of same-sex partners and implications for next of kin in relation to health service provision. Some spoke about their actual experiences in this regard and the issue most commonly raised was the importance of the recognition of same-sex partnerships, especially when an LGB client is hospitalised or wishes to become a parent. Respondents expressed concerns about whether they would be: entitled to access information on their partner's health; allowed visiting access; and involved in decision-making with their partner in the case of serious health issues. A number of women also raised more general concerns regarding their treatment as lesbians if they decide to have a child in the future. These concerns were highlighted in the context of a lack of legal recognition of same-sex relationships.

Mental Health

Almost all respondents referred to mental health as a central issue in the health care of LGB people. The experiences of respondents who accessed mental health services because of emotional or psychological distress varied. Many sought support for problems associated with their sexual identity but this was not the case for all. Generally, interviewees stressed the need for mental health professionals to offer a welcoming, listening space and to have sensitivity to all the issues involved. Even supportive service providers were not always felt to have an understanding of the particular experiences of LGB clients and the impact of heterosexism on their lives.

Sexual/Gynaecological Health

Sexual health was identified by a majority of the participants in this study as a key issue for LGB people. Overall, the male respondents were primarily concerned with the provision of gay-friendly sexual health services, while women stressed the need for gynaecological health services that are appropriate for lesbians. Some of the interviewees were critical of the lack of knowledge amongst health care providers and amongst the lesbian population concerning the general sexual/gynaecological health of lesbians. The data suggests that doctors and nurses in this field require comprehensive awareness training around the health and service-related needs of their lesbian clients. Moreover, confidentiality was a significant concern in relation to sexual health matters, particularly given the rural nature of the north west region.

Suggestions for Improved Health Services for LGB Clients

Throughout the interviews participants made many suggestions about how services could be improved in order to enhance the experience of LGB clients using health services. The following summary draws these suggestions together, grouping in sequence the proposed specific actions for the health system generally, for all health care providers, for particular service settings and finally for LGB people themselves.

For the organisation	◦ Emphasise a culture of 'equal rights' rather than 'special treatment'.
	◦ Counter heterosexism and homophobia throughout the organisation.
	◦ Acknowledge that both service users and staff may be LGB and raise the visibility of the group throughout the health service.
	◦ Introduce and influence more training on LGB issues and the social context and on medical issues specific to LGB patients.
	◦ Form partnerships with the LGB community.
	◦ Work proactively with the education sector.
	◦ Address issues of same-sex partners and next of kin in health care settings.
For all service providers	◦ Seek and secure training about LGB issues and perspectives and about specific medical issues for LGB people.
	◦ Do not assume clients are heterosexual; be more accepting of difference.
	◦ If an LGB client decides to disclose her/his sexual identity, react appropriately.
	◦ Be sensitive to what stage an LGB client is at in the process of 'coming out'.
For all service settings	◦ Improve confidentiality and privacy.
	◦ Disseminate appropriate information, particularly for young LGB people.
For particular services	◦ Understand and meet the needs of LGB people in sexual health services.
	◦ Understand and meet the needs of LGB people in mental health services.
	◦ Understand and meet the needs of LGB people in GP services.
For LGB people	◦ Take more responsibility for setting the context with the service provider.
	◦ Collect relevant local information and supply it to service providers.

1

INTRODUCTION AND CONTEXT

HSE West,[1] through its Department of Public Health and Equality Office, received funding from the Equality Authority to research and document the experiences of lesbian, gay and bisexual (LGB)[2] people with the health services in the north west region. This report is the culmination of that research.

Drawing upon the personal testimony of a sample of 43 lesbian, gay or bisexual respondents, obtained through in-depth interviews, this report explores their experiences as health service users and their perspectives on the quality of care that they receive. In documenting this lived experience, it illuminates the barriers that restrict LGB people from accessing the health services on an equal footing and discusses how these barriers can be addressed and how good practice can be encouraged at the level of the HSE and of the individual service providers. Throughout, it aims to enable the voice of the participant to be fully heard. As such it represents an important step in countering the invisibility and silence of the LGB community in the health services as well as in wider society.

The co-ordinating team for this study comprised Caoimhe Gleeson, Equality Officer and Dr Mary Manandhar, Department of Public Health, HSE West. The members of the research team were Dr Maria Gibbons, Independent Researcher; and Dr Mary Manandhar and Joan Mullan, Department of Public Health, HSE West. An Advisory Group was formed at the outset to advise the researchers in defining the research aims and to guide both research design and the research process. In order to ensure participation and empowerment of the lesbian, gay and bisexual community through the research process, this Advisory Group included members of the LGB community as well as HSE West area staff.[3] Advice was also sought from two external experts[4] on qualitative research methodologies, sexual orientation and health issues, and health-care-seeking behaviour.

---

[1] This research was undertaken through the North Western Health Board (NWHB) prior to the establishment of the Health Service Executive (HSE). The former NWHB, which operated in the counties of Donegal, Sligo, Leitrim and west Cavan, now forms part of the HSE West administrative area. This research relates only to the administrative boundaries of the former NWHB.

[2] Transgender people are commonly included in considerations of lesbian, gay and bisexual issues (giving rise to the abbreviation LGBT). However, this research does not include transgender people's experiences and refers to the experiences of lesbian, gay and bisexual people only.

[3] The Advisory Group members were Ruth Charlton, Representative of Lesbian Community, Sligo/Leitrim; Martin Cooke, Representative of Gay Community, Sligo/Leitrim; Representative of Gay Community, Donegal (six months only – name withheld by request); Michael McMonigle, Community Worker, Children Services, Representative of Men's Health, HSE West.

[4] Ursula Barry of University College Dublin; Dr Alizon Draper of the University of Westminster, London, UK.

This introductory chapter briefly outlines the social and policy context for the study and sets out the aims of the research. The study approach and the key themes are addressed in Chapter 2.

1.1 Social Context

Considerable progress has been made by LGB people in Ireland in addressing prejudice and discrimination based on sexual orientation (Equality Authority, 2002). In addition to building a wide variety of community supports, including activist and social organisations, LGB people have been to the fore in contributing to far-reaching legislative and policy change, including equality legislation and the decriminalisation of homosexuality.

The Employment Equality Acts 1998 and 2007 prohibit discrimination in the workplace and in vocational training. The Equal Status Acts 2000 to 2004 prohibit discrimination in the provision of goods and services, accommodation and education. Both Acts cover nine grounds including the ground of sexual orientation. The Equal Status Acts cover the provision of goods and services, accommodation and education by the public sector including the provision of health services. Both Acts contain a number of exemptions.

Despite such legal developments, it is essential to recognise that discrimination against LGB people still widely exists as a socially acceptable and institutionally sanctioned form of prejudice (Snape et al., 1995; GLEN and Nexus Research Cooperative, 1995; Equality Authority, 2002; Huebner et al., 2002). Furthermore, many people continue to hide or deny their LGB sexual identity to avoid facing discrimination in several areas of their lives (Combat Poverty Agency and Equality Authority, 2003).

Discrimination against LGB people can result from heterosexism and/or homophobia. Heterosexism is the process and consequences of the socially embedded assumption that all people are heterosexual, which stems from a belief that heterosexuality is the only 'normal' or 'natural' form of sexuality and that heterosexuality is thus the only valid sexual orientation (Quiery, 2002; Cooper, 1994). This has resulted in heterosexuality being privileged legally, culturally, educationally, socially and economically.

Heterosexism is so pervasive that it is hard to recognise and identify, let alone deal with (Trotter, 1999). The assumption of heterosexuality is so prevalent that health care providers may perpetuate the invisibility of the LGB experience and discriminate against those who are in same-sex relationships (Denenberg, 1995; Rankow, 1995; Dibble et al., 2002). An emerging body of research is attempting to describe and address the problems associated with LGB invisibility in order to meet the health care needs of this population (Albarran and Salmon, 2000).

Homophobia is the fear and/or hatred of homosexuality and of gay men and lesbians. Homophobia can be expressed at an individual level as harassment, bullying and hate crime. It can also be expressed at an institutional level as direct or indirect discrimination (Herek and Berrill, 1992; Trotter, 1999; Quiery, 2002; Jarman and Tennant, 2003; Hickson et al., 2003; Norman et al., 2006).

Homophobia or anti-homosexual bias can also result in LGB people experiencing negative feelings towards themselves when they first recognise their differing identity in adolescence or adulthood. This is referred to as internalised homophobia and it can make the process of 'coming out' more difficult for LGB people. A higher level of internalised homophobia is associated with greater psychological distress, lower self-esteem, lower levels of self-disclosure about one's sexual orientation and also reduced social support (Herek et al., 1998).

Societal and individual discrimination against LGB people, and the resultant social exclusion and marginalisation of LGB people, are the crucial contexts within which the pathways and potential barriers to LGB people accessing and receiving appropriate and good quality health care must be understood.

1.2 Sexual Orientation and National Health Policy

The amount of national, regional and local policy addressing sexual orientation and the LGB population has been increasing in recent years. The last decade has witnessed the production of major strategic, advocacy, policy and research documents on LGB issues, particularly around identity, education and health (O'Carroll and Collins, 1995; Wardlaw, 1994; Taillon, 1999; O'Carroll, 1999; Dillon, 1999; Dillon and Collins, 2004; Gay HIV Strategies et al., 1999; Gay HIV Strategies and

Nexus Research Cooperative, 2000; GLEN and Nexus Research Cooperative, 1995; Mee and Ronayne, 2000; Equality Authority, 2002; NESF, 2003; Carolan and Redmond, 2003; Barron and Collins, 2005; BeLonG To, 2005; Working Group on Domestic Partnership, 2006; Norman *et al.,* 2006; Sarma, 2007). Despite this changing policy situation, the equality ground of sexual orientation still remains one of the least evident on the agendas of public services, community and voluntary services and private sector bodies. This invisibility is compounded particularly where rural communities predominate, as in the north west of Ireland.

In relation to health and health care, LGB people are still not a named group in many key health policy documents at national and regional levels. Existing literature on the issue of health and well-being within the LGB community has tended to focus on the issue of HIV/AIDS. As a result of the concentration on gay men and HIV/AIDS, there has been a deficit in work around other health issues in the LGB community, particularly lesbian health. However, in recent years there have been some notable developments. For example *A Plan for Women's Health* (DOHC, 1997) highlighted lesbian health issues as a major concern and *The National Health Promotion Strategy 2000–2005* (DOHC, 2000) noted the particular needs of lesbians and gay men.

In 2002 the Equality Authority's strategic document *Implementing Equality for Lesbians, Gays and Bisexuals* included specific recommendations for health and the LGB community. In *Equality Policies for Lesbian, Gay and Bisexual People: Implementation Issues* (2003), the National Economic and Social Forum (NESF) examined the issues raised in the Equality Authority report. While noting that there had been positive developments, particularly in the area of HIV/AIDS for men, the NESF found a lack of visibility of LGB issues within the health system. It recommended that this should be addressed to a greater degree and made specific recommendations regarding the particular concerns of LGB people. These issues were taken up by the Department of Health and Children which, in a December 2002 Circular, urged action to implement the NESF issues (DOHC, 2002). The Department of Justice, Equality and Law Reform is now working together with GLEN to stimulate and support the implementation of the NESF recommendations by government departments.

A Vision for Change, Report of the Expert Group on Mental Health Policy, which has been adopted as the Department of Health and Children's mental health policy, refers to the fact that 'there is a small but significant number of people in Ireland who have additional needs when they develop a mental health problem' (DOHC, 2006: 40) including gay and lesbian individuals (among others). The report also identifies 'same-sex' attraction as a suicide risk factor.

Reach-Out, the government's ten-year strategy on suicide prevention, names LGBT people as a marginalised group with particular vulnerability. The strategy recommends that the HSE, as a suicide prevention measure, should promote research and services to support LGBT people (HSE and DOHC, 2005).

Two recent health policy documents have made explicit reference to equality and LGB people. *Equal Status Acts and the Provision of Health Services,* published in 2005, sets out the HSE's responsibilities to all patients/service users under the Equal Status Acts 2000 to 2004 and specifically includes LGB people (Equality Authority, HSE and DOHC, 2005). *Get Connected – Developing an Adolescent Friendly Health Service* indicates that 'there should be an increased focus on the health needs of adolescents who are members of minority groups with the emphasis being placed on equality and discrimination issues' (DOHC, 2001: 83). It further recommends that every public service should have a policy and protocol in response to the needs of gay and lesbian adolescents.

1.3 Local Context

The north west region, comprising Donegal, Sligo, Leitrim and west Cavan, is a predominantly rural area with limited social infrastructure to support the LGB community.

The experiences of LGB people in relation to health services in the region are undocumented and under-explored. However, in terms of activities around sexual orientation, there have been important local developments and activities in relation to LGB issues since 1999. These include:

- North West Lesbian Line (a confidential telephone service which provides information and support to women questioning their sexuality in the north west and border areas).

- Women Out And About Support Group (an informal social group in the Sligo area which organises social, educational and health-related events for lesbian and bisexual women in the north west region).
- OutWest (a support group for LGB men and women in the west and north west areas).
- Gay Men's Helpline (a confidential telephone service which provides information and support to gay and bisexual men in the north west and west areas).
- North West Pride (an annual parade and associated events to highlight issues of visibility and inclusion of LGBT people throughout the north west region).

The implementation of these activities has increased the organisational capacity of the LGB community in the region. Specific actions have also been included in the multiagency strategic plans of the Sligo and Leitrim County Development Boards (for the period from 2002 to 2012) that aim to break the silence on hidden issues related to health, including access to services, experienced by the LGB community.

1.4 Study Aims

Given the evolving national and local context outlined above, this research was stimulated by several factors:

- The perception that there are considerable numbers of LGB people living in the north west, many of whom are not 'out' (or who do not openly identify themselves to the wider community as lesbian, gay or bisexual), and about whom the health system still knows very little.
- Concerns expressed by the local LGB community regarding their experience of health services.
- A growing body of evidence, nationally and internationally, that the LGB community experiences inequities in health services, with detrimental effects on their health and well-being.

The study was designed to explore the following questions:

- What are the experiences of LGB people living in the HSE West region in relation to health services?
- Are these services meeting the needs of LGB clients?
- Do LGB clients experience any difficulties?
- If yes, what is the nature and the extent of these difficulties and how can they be addressed and overcome?
- How can good practice be encouraged and replicated?

2

STUDY APPROACH AND KEY THEMES

This study uses qualitative methods to record the experiences of LGB people in accessing health services in the north west region. This chapter describes the research approach, participation in the study and the key themes and structure of the report. It begins by introducing some of the terminology used throughout this report.

2.1 Terminology

The term 'gay' refers to a person whose primary sexual attraction is to people of the same sex. The term is most commonly applied to men who self-identify as same sex attracted. While many women identify as gay, the term 'lesbian' is commonly used to describe same-sex-attracted women. The term 'bisexual' refers to a person who is sexually attracted to people of both sexes. In this study, participants described themselves in the main as lesbian, gay or bisexual. The abbreviation 'LGB' will be utilised to describe the common sexual identity of participants. The abbreviation 'LGBT', which includes transgender people, will be used only in reference to other studies.

The terms 'LGB sexual orientation', 'LGB sexual identity' and 'LGB sexuality' were used interchangeably by participants throughout the interviews and will be used interchangeably throughout this report. Participants frequently used the terms 'coming out' and 'out' to describe the process of acknowledging one's LGB sexual orientation and telling (or disclosing it to) other people, friends, family, colleagues at work and society at large. Participants used the terms 'closet' and 'closeted' to describe the process of hiding one's sexual orientation and not telling other people, friends, family, colleagues at work and society at large.

The terms 'client', 'patient' and 'service user' will be used interchangeably in reference to LGB people who use health services.

2.2 Recruiting Participants

Initially participants were sought through an extensive publicity campaign.[5] Any lesbian, gay or bisexual person over the age of 18 years living in the north west region (Counties Sligo, Leitrim,

---

[5] This campaign targeted over thirty national, regional and local newspapers and six local radio stations during spring and summer 2003. Email was also used to circulate information to national magazines, organisations, websites and community groups and four presentations were made to LGB community groups. Information on the research was widely circulated in the north west region and a flier was also sent to every GP surgery in the region with a request to display the information in the surgery waiting area.

Donegal and west Cavan), or who had until recently been living in the region, and who had used the health services of the HSE West in the previous ten years was eligible to participate in the study. The researchers followed up contact from people expressing an interest in participating. They provided information on the study including details of the research process and how issues of confidentiality and safety would be addressed. Not all of those who initially made contact agreed to be interviewed. While most of the men interviewed volunteered in response to the publicity campaign, only one woman was recruited through this method. Thus, most of the women interviewed were recruited via subsequent snowballing contacts through lesbian organisations mainly in the Sligo/Leitrim area.

The difficulty recruiting study participants is a common challenge for research in this area (McManus, 2003). It underlines the challenges presented in trying to assess and meet the health and health care needs of the LGB population. Based on evidence from elsewhere and concerns identified by the research participants, these difficulties reflect the hidden nature of the LGB population and its health needs and the fears of this population about discrimination, prejudice and homophobia (Hall, 1999).

The individual interviews reveal a consistency in the data in terms of the concerns and experiences of many participants in relation to their use of health-related services. Nevertheless, recruitment issues are likely to have impacted on at least some of the results obtained. In particular, most women who participated were connected to the lesbian community in the Sligo area, where there is an informal lesbian support network. While men who took part in the study were generally less networked within a gay community than the women were, overall most participants – women and men – were 'out' to some degree, both in terms of their own self-acknowledgement and comfort and of disclosure to many people around them. Thus, the acceptance and positive view of LGB sexuality observed among participants, although welcome, may in part be a function of the recruitment process and not fully reflective of the experience of the wider LGB population and this factor must be kept in mind when reading the report.

2.3 Conducting Interviews

The interviews were undertaken between September and December 2003. Interviews were held at a time and place that suited the participant, generally in the participant's home, a local hotel or in a discreet HSE West venue.

A member of the lesbian community who is also a researcher conducted all of the interviews. The matching of sexuality between interviewees and interviewer was considered important to enhancing trust, empathy and feelings of empowerment for interviewees. Initially the intention was to use an interviewer from the gay men's community to interview men in the study. However, no such interviewer became available for the purposes of the study. There has been discussion about the need to match the sexual orientation of interviewers with study participants in research on sexual-identity-related research (McManus, 2003) and the appropriateness of disclosure of information about an interviewer in the research process (Ndofor-Tah *et al.,* 2000). Matching has been a feature of many studies undertaken about the experiences of LGB people and some authors argue strongly for matching in all aspects of the research process (Bradford *et al.,* 2001).

These one-to-one interviews lasted between 1 and 2.5 hours. The topic guide for the interviews was informed by key issues highlighted in the literature and by the recommendations of the Advisory Group and external advisers. It included a series of questions covering use of health-related services, experience of services, attitudes towards services and role and/or impact of LGB sexuality on use of services. A semi-structured approach was used in questioning and probing prompts were included. A checklist of HSE and other health-related services used by the participant within the previous ten years was completed by each participant during the early stages of the interview. Participants were also asked to complete a data sheet requesting demographic and other background information.

Interviews were audio-taped and transcribed. The interviewer, a project co-ordinator and an external company[6] transcribed the interviews. A thematic analysis was undertaken on the interview transcripts. Each transcript was indexed and its content coded. The broad framework for analysis was arrived at in a participatory manner through discussion with the research advisory group. Drafts of results were

---

[6] The external company was only used after the prior agreement of the participant had been obtained. This company had agreed standards of confidentiality.

circulated to and discussed with research participants to check the validity of findings from their perspective and to ensure participants were satisfied with the manner in which their information had been used.

2.4 Ethical Issues

At the time of the study design, there were no specific in-house policies for conducting ethical community-based research in the then NWHB.[7] However, the principles of socially responsible and ethical good practice in conducting health-related research were adhered to in this study (CIOMS, 1993; Nuffield Council on Bioethics, 2002; World Medical Association, 2004). These were:

- To provide clear information prior to and at the time of interview and during dissemination.
- To obtain consent and allow time for reflection, questions and refusals.
- To state the benefits of the research for various parties involved.
- To deal with people respectfully and with cultural sensitivity.

The fullest possible information about the rationale, aims, methods and expected outcomes of the research was included in publicity about the study. At the time of interview, participants were informed about plans for use and dissemination of the research findings. They were told that they would be invited to a dissemination event, would receive a copy of the final report and were given an opportunity to ask questions. An information pack was supplied to each participant, which included contact details of support groups in the area and other LGB-related material.

The research team followed a rigorous procedure for obtaining consent. Participants gave their signed consent to be interviewed. Permission was sought to tape-record each interview. Participants were informed of their right to withdraw from the study at any stage, even after being interviewed. Each participant was provided with a confidentiality statement, which had been discussed with participants prior to interview. A written commitment was made to return to each participant their tape recording as well as a hard copy of the transcript of their interview; this would allow them to verify the accuracy of the data collected and would serve as a reference in validating the final document.

Sensitivity is required in probing intimate and sometimes disturbing aspects of an individual's life (Eth, 1992). A trained therapist advised the project on how issues arising for participants might be handled. After the interviews, a project co-ordinator telephoned each participant to thank them for taking part and to inform them of the next steps for the project. Additionally, particular sensitivity was paid throughout the research to the disempowerment and social exclusion experienced by many LGB people and also to the dynamics of the power differences between interviewers and those being interviewed (Adamson and Donovan, 2002).

2.5 Participation in the Study

The initial target was to carry out 48 interviews and to achieve a diverse sample in terms of gender, age group (under and over 40 years old), area of residence (rural/urban) and degree of being 'out' as an LGB person. In fact 43 interviews were completed, of which 24 were with women and 19 with men (see Table 2.1); 27 participants were aged under 40 and 16 were 40 or older. There were 22 urban and 21 rural participants; 25 lived in County Sligo, ten in County Donegal and six in County Leitrim. Two of those interviewed were from the region but were living outside it at the time of interview.

In the interviews the vast majority of participants identified themselves as lesbian (women) or as gay (men). One interviewee, a man, identified himself primarily as bisexual,[8] and four self-described lesbians also saw themselves somewhere on a continuum between being lesbian and heterosexual. One interviewee identified as a gay male transvestite.[9] Participants reported that they had self-identified as lesbian or gay for two years to over thirty years and "as far back as I can remember". Male participants tended to be 'out' in terms of their gay identity for longer than women participants.

---

[7] The situation has since changed as membership of the Research Ethics Committee has been expanded in order to cover community-based research of a quantitative as well as a qualitative nature.

[8] In order to protect his identity, quotes relating to his experience are included throughout the document but he is not separately named as bisexual.

[9] A transvestite is defined as someone who cross-dresses with the desire to adopt the clothes, appearance and behaviour associated with the opposite gender.

Table 2.1: Profile of Participants

		Women	Men	All
All		24	19	43
Age group	18–39	13	14	27
	40+	11	5	16
County	Leitrim	3	3	6
	Sligo	16	9	25
	Donegal	3	7	10
	Other	2	0	2
Urban/rural	Urban	12	10	22
	Rural	12	9	21

Twenty-five interviewees were not in a relationship at the time of interview. Eighteen participants were in a relationship with a same-sex partner and 16 were living with these partners. Two participants were in a relationship with an opposite-sex partner. Four men and three women were, or had been, married at some stage and six participants were parents of a dependent child.

2.6 Sexual Identity and Use of Health Services

While participants had experience of a wide range of HSE West's services, they asserted that LGB sexual identity was more relevant to some services than others. This was the case where the nature of the service meant that sexual orientation was more likely to arise as an issue for the client.

The most widely used service was the general practitioner (GP) service – everyone had attended a GP at some point. All participants acknowledged that the issue of sexual orientation might arise at some stage in interactions with GP services. The areas of sexual health and mental health were regarded as being particularly relevant to their GP health care as LGB clients. Also mentioned in this regard were issues relating to next of kin, maternity/parenting, gynaecological health and blood-testing. See Appendix, Table A1.

Nine participants had been hospitalised in acute hospitals in the region and four had spent time in acute hospitals elsewhere. One respondent had direct dealings with hospitals both locally and outside the region due to the illness of her partner. However the issue of hospitalisation came up in almost half of the interviews (n=20), and was linked by participants to LGB sexual identity in all but three cases. Almost all of these interviewees raised concerns about how next of kin/partnership issues are dealt with in hospitals. See Appendix, Table A2.

Twenty-four participants attended hospital emergency departments during the study period. In the minority of instances where sexual orientation arose (n=7), it was usually in relation to assumptions made by staff that the client was heterosexual, or partnership issues.

The vast majority of respondents felt that mental and sexual health services have particular significance for LGB clients. All nine of the men who attended mental health professionals (excluding GPs) identified their sexuality as being at least partly relevant to their consultations, as did five of the 13 women. In addition, most of the remaining interviewees referred to LGB people as having specific mental health needs from health services. See Appendix, Table A3.

Among the participants, two men had attended the Sligo genito-urinary medicine (GUM) clinic, six other men had visited a GUM clinic elsewhere, and no woman reported visiting a GUM clinic. All of the men and two-thirds of the women interviewed brought up issues of LGB sexuality in relation to sexual/gynaecological health and sexual health services, generally during the course of the interview.

No interviewee attended maternity services in the region during the study period. One woman went to a fertility clinic in London and another used the maternity services in Dublin during that time. However, obstetrical health was relevant for six lesbians who expressed a desire to bear children. Almost all of these women considered the undertaking with concerns regarding how their same-sex partners would be treated within the health system, especially in relation to GPs and hospital maternity services.

Complementary health services were accessed by almost half of the interviewees (n= 21) during the study period.[10] The majority of these were lesbians (n=15). A total of 14 out of the 21 interviewees who attended complementary services stated that the issue of their sexual identity arose at some stage during the treatment. This was particularly the case for women rather than men.[11]

There are some services where issues associated with sexual identity arose for a small proportion of participants. These include the pharmacy service, dental service, X-ray department, hospital outpatients department, community welfare officer, home help, men's health officer within the specialised sexual health services, social work service and the Blood Transfusion Service Board. There are also many other health services where participants reported that sexual identity did not arise for them and where they considered it unlikely to become relevant at any stage. These include the ambulance service, most administrative services and many routine hospital departments such as orthopaedics, paediatrics and ENT.

2.7 Key Themes and Structure of the Report

A number of key themes emerged from the study and guided the structure of this report. Most of these themes arose across more than one service, although some emerged more frequently in respect to particular specialities than others. The main themes arising from the study can be categorised as:

- **Disclosure of sexual orientation.** The disclosure, or not, of LGB sexual identity to service providers appeared to be a significant factor influencing health care for interviewees. Anxieties concerning confidentiality, homophobia and heterosexism emerged across all the services in this regard.
- **Recognition of partnerships/next of kin.** Concerns with regard to partnership rights, particularly in relation to hospitalisation and GP services.
- **Parenthood.** Arose primarily for women in relation to GP and maternity services.
- **Mental health.** Primarily arose in relation to GPs and other mental health professionals.
- **Sexual/gynaecological health.** Arose mainly in relation to GPs and other sexual health professionals.
- **Suggestions for improvements.** Interviewees made many recommendations towards improving the health services for LGB clients. These applied across all of the services.

Chapter 3 provides an overview of the important national and international research literature that is relevant to the question of LGB people and access to health services.

Chapter 4 examines what the interviews tell us about the experiences of respondents with regards to living as a lesbian, gay or bisexual person in the north west of Ireland.

Chapters 5 to 9 construct an in-depth picture of the experiences of LGB people in their use of health services in the north west. One of the key themes addressed by participants in the study is disclosure of LGB sexual orientation to health service providers. This emerged as an overarching theme linked to all the other themes that arose in the research. Chapter 5 looks at the broad factors influencing disclosure of lesbian, gay or bisexual sexual identity in accessing health services and Chapter 6 examines the experiences of disclosure of LGB sexual orientation specifically in relation to GP services. Chapter 7 addresses issues relating to recognition of same-sex partners and LGB parenthood. Chapters 8 and 9 discuss mental health issues and sexual and gynaecological health issues respectively.

The remaining chapters consider how improvements in the quality of health care that is available to LGB people in the north west can be achieved. Chapter 10 offers a range of recommendations suggested directly by the research participants. These are intended to help deliver practical improvements in the service supplied by both the HSE and individual health professionals, making it more appropriate to the needs of LGB people. Chapter 11 restates the fundamental issues that are relevant to the experiences of LGB people in the north west and summarises the core recommendations for change that emerged from the research.

---

[10] These services included chiropractic, reflexology, massage and acupuncture services.
[11] Thirteen out of the 15 women stated that sexual identity arose as an issue at some stage in their attendance at complementary practitioners, while this was the case for only one of the six men.

3

LITERATURE REVIEW

There is a growing body of evidence, nationally and internationally, showing that LGB people experience inequities in access to and contact with health services, and that these inequities, and the social context in which they are embedded, can have detrimental effects on their health and well-being. This chapter reviews the available research literature on the issues related to access to health services for LGB people. Firstly it examines the dynamics of the relationships between service users and health service professionals and explores how these relationships can be more fraught for LGB people. The next section offers an overview of the central importance that the issue of disclosure of sexuality plays for LGB people concerning the level of trust they develop with their health care providers and the quality of care that they receive. Following this, the question of the lack of recognition of same-sex partners as authentic family support networks within health care settings is discussed. The literature review then presents an overview of the core issues relating to access to primary care, mental health and other health services for LGB people. The chapter concludes by analysing the importance of health personnel in the debate and briefly engaging with the question of how health systems accommodate staff members who are lesbian, gay or bisexual.

3.1 LGB Client–Service Provider Interface

> It's hard to feel comfortable and in control of your health care process.
> (An American lesbian in a primary care setting, Diamant *et al.,* 2000a)

The face-to-face interaction of client and provider lies at the core of the health system and the provision of health care. The dynamics of this relationship, together with learned experience through their previous encounters or those of trusted others, determines to a large degree clients' access to health care (Stevens, 1998). Comprehensive health care depends in part on the quality of the relationship between the service provider and the patient. The degree of trust in the service provider has been correlated with the number of health care visits and with therapeutic outcomes (Smith *et al.,* 1985).

The client–service provider relationship is hierarchical in nature with greater power going to the service provider, who generally controls questioning and activities within the encounter (Klitzman and Greenberg, 2002). Service providers may not be aware of or experience this power differential in transactions but it may be strongly felt by clients (Stevens, 1998). The imbalance may be more profound when clients come from less socially privileged groups (Stevens, 1998).

Little is documented or known about the interface between LGB clients and health care providers and how the dynamics and processes of this relationship can impact on access to the service, on quality of care received, and ultimately on health outcomes for the client. In Boehmer's (2002) review of 20 years of published research into LGB health, only 5.5% (n=207) of the 3,777 articles reviewed had explored providers' attitudes and cultural competency, patient–provider relationships and LGB people's experiences with health service delivery.

Work in the area of LGB people's access to health services has mainly been around primary care in relation to general practitioners (GPs), social services such as social work, nursing care, sexual health and mental health services. Most of the evidence is from North America, although a body of work is now growing in the UK. The Scottish LGBT Health Project, which is run under the auspices of Stonewall Scotland, gathered data on LGBT people's experiences of NHS services (Pringle, 2003; Miller, 2003). This research led to the establishment of demonstration sites to look at how knowledge and awareness of LGBT people's needs can be improved and how the UK National Health Service (NHS) can ensure that LGBT people's experiences of the service, as patients and employees, are enhanced (Miller, 2003).

Evidence suggests that LGB people make greater use of services where identified 'gay-friendly' services exist, particularly in relation to sexual and mental health issues (Ginsburg et al., 2002). Where services have attempted to cater for the specific requirements of LGB people, there has been a greater use of the service, a higher satisfaction level and also health gain (Turner and Mallett, 1998).

3.2 Disclosure of LGB Sexual Identity in Health Care Settings

The process of disclosing sexuality appears to play a crucial role in the health and well-being of LGB people but disclosing oneself as LGB is rarely easy. Most gay men and lesbians perceive self-disclosure as a risk (Franke and Leary, 1991; Dillon and Collins, 2004) and emphasise vigilance, safety and self-protection (Hitchcock and Wilson, 1992). Fears held by LGB people about potential negative effects of disclosure are well documented (Rose, 1993; Saddul, 1996). Failure to disclose non-heterosexual orientation has been described as 'wearing a mask as a survival technique' (White and Martinez, 1997). Cain (1991) argues that subtle heterosexist bias in the health system and among individual service providers can make it difficult to disclose LGB sexuality. In Van Voorhis and Wagner's review (2002) of LGB people in social work research, disclosure of sexual orientation emerged as the second – after HIV/AIDS – most commonly reported and problematic component for LGB people in consulting a health care professional or gaining access to treatment. This non-disclosure can be perceived as a sign of not having accepted one's homosexual identity. An understanding of the role of 'outness' in the lives of LGB people therefore has important implications, especially for mental health (Bradford et al., 1994).

With the use of tools[12] to evaluate negative beliefs and attitudes towards LGB people and the existence of homophobia (Eliason, 2000), evidence emerges of homophobia by some health care providers in the delivery of care to LGB patients (Greco and Glusman, 1998; Wells, 1997; Klitzman and Greenberg, 2002). Many LGB people do not reveal their sexual orientation to their GP through fear of homophobia and/or breach of confidentiality and too often providers are afraid to broach the subject of sexual identity with LGB people (Carr, 1999). Ginsburg et al. (2002) describe how LGB people have heard others label LGB people as deviant, and many may choose to remain quiet rather than face rejection and abuse (Diamant and Wold, 2003). Even when asked by their physicians, patients do not always accurately disclose their sexual orientation, and Klitzman and Greenberg (2002) found that the vast majority of lesbians imagine their care will be less if they disclose.

Irish research has also reported that negative experiences cause lesbians to hide their sexual identity from various service providers because of fear of prejudice and discrimination (Rose, 1998; L.Inc, 2006). During the consultation process preceding the publication of *A Plan for Women's Health* (DOHC, 1997), the most serious health issue identified by lesbian participants nationwide was the negative attitudes that they encountered when seeking care from the health services (Women's Health Council, 2003).

---

[12] Such as the Attitudes Towards Lesbians and Gays (ATLG) questionnaire (Herek, 1994).

The beliefs, attitudes and values of health care professionals may have a profound impact on the treatment that LGB people receive (Berkman and Zinberg, 1997; Eliason, 2000) and can lead to situations where LGB people are effectively invisible within the health care setting with the result that their needs may not be appropriately met. There is evidence of reduced nurse contact, a change of demeanour, less professionally initiated verbal interactions and distancing by providers following client disclosure of LGB sexual orientation, as well as behaviours such as leaving the room or refusing to be involved in the care of patients they perceive to be 'perverts' (Walpin, 1997; Stewart, 1999; Ginsburg *et al.,* 2002). Conversely, sometimes lesbians and gay men can be the subject of almost voyeuristic attention (Rose and Platzer, 1993; Stevens, 1995).

Smith (1992) argues that prejudicial stereotyping means that practitioners will ignore, or be unable to obtain, information that may be relevant to the LGB patient's treatment or delivery of care. Prejudicial attitudes expressed towards LGB people will also inhibit the ability to convey empathy and human concern (Klitzman and Greenberg, 2002; Pringle, 2003). Research evidence has illustrated the negative impact of sexual identity stereotyping on patients (Holyoake, 1999; Johnson and Webb, 1995; Morrisey, 1996; Wilton, 1999). In a US study of LGB youths, participants described what they regarded as positive features in a service provider (e.g. clinicians being educated about their lifestyle) and what offended them (e.g. equating their sexuality with HIV). In the area of mental health, negative internalised stereotypes held by gay people about their own sexuality may be reinforced by therapists who also hold these stereotypes and who do not recognise that they are symptomatic of homophobia (US Committee on Human Sexuality, 2000; APA, 2000). Satisfaction with health care has been found to be greater among gay men and lesbians who disclosed their sexual orientation (Smith *et al.,* 1985).

The issue of trust is central to disclosure of sexual orientation. Many authors suggest that building a client–provider relationship in which LGB sexuality is acknowledged and unconditionally accepted is essential to building an atmosphere of trust (Albarran and Salmon, 2000). Such an atmosphere of trust and acceptance can also facilitate disclosure of information that may be sensitive but important in dealing with health issues (Klitzman and Greenberg, 2002). Confidentiality is a major concern for many LGB people in terms of what information is recorded on medical records and who might see those records (Klitzman and Greenberg, 2002). The need to have certainty about confidentiality and an awareness of what happens to information is also essential to building an atmosphere of trust that will support LGB clients in disclosing their sexuality if they consider it to be important. Simple measures such as service providers stating during consultations that information provided will be confidential have been suggested (Ginsburg *et al.,* 2002).

3.3 LGB Familial and Social Support Networks

Another key issue emerging from the literature is the lack of recognition of LGB relationships as authentic family support networks. Many LGB people face rejection or the possibility of rejection from families, and as a result they often form strong emotional bonds with other members of LGB networks to replace lost family support (Eliason, 2000; APA, 2000). Although these significant people become like family members, in many situations they are not included in the treatment process and are even excluded from visiting access. The same experience also extends to same-sex partners (Equality Authority, 2002). This situation can place enormous additional emotional strain on LGB patients already in vulnerable physical and emotional states. In Canada, Albarran and Salmon (2000) identified the emotionally distressing and traumatic effects of disclosure for many LGB people in critical care, a setting in which all patients and the people close to them experience heightened vulnerability. When a patient's condition is serious, those closest to the patient, in particular the patient's partner, will be essential in providing information for the purposes of planning care.

Dibble *et al.* (2002), discussing the matter in a nursing context, suggest that the approach undertaken to questioning can signal to LGB clients, their family and friends that sharing information about their lives is safe. This can include, for example, asking whether a client would like a partner or friend to participate in a consultation about their health. The American Psychological Association (2000) recommends that clients be asked who constitutes their significant 'family' members and who they would like to have involved in their care. The outcome of such approaches is to enable the practitioner to provide better care.

3.4 LGB People and Primary Care

Appropriate and high-quality initial consultations and referrals are essential to the health care of all people, including those in the LGB population group (Brotman *et al.,* 2002; Mathieson *et al.,* 2002). The evidence overall indicates a general problem of delay and avoidance accessing preventative primary care in the LGB population and a range of still poorly understood and unmet needs (Boehmer, 2002). Harrison and Silenzio (1996) suggest that the most significant health risk for LGB people is that of avoiding routine medical examinations that can help prevent and reduce serious medical illness through early detection.

Diamant *et al.* (2000a, 2000b) report that 89% of lesbians and bisexual women had a negative reaction when they 'came out' to their doctor, ranging from embarrassment to inappropriate questions, coolness and rejection. A Canadian study of family practice physicians found that over one-third had scores on an attitude test that reflected homophobic views, although only 23% admitted that they were prejudiced against LGB people (Chaimowitz, 1991).

Evidence suggests that there are health benefits for patients who disclose their LGB sexual identity to their GP. For example, in a study on HIV-negative men, the incidence of cancers and moderately serious infection was directly proportional to the degree of non-disclosure of sexual orientation – the more closeted the individual, the more susceptible he was to developing such conditions (Brotman *et al.,* 2002). Doctors are able to give more appropriate advice to men whom they know to be gay. The available evidence also strongly suggests that having a gay-friendly doctor greatly facilitates open communication about substance use, high-risk sexual behaviour, mental health issues and other important health topics (Klitzman and Greenberg, 2002).

In New York, a study exploring patterns of communication between 94 gay and lesbian patients and their health care providers in the primary care setting found that men were more likely than women to disclose their sexual orientation, to feel comfortable discussing sex and to have a male doctor (Klitzman and Greenberg, 2002).

3.5 LGB People and Mental Health/Emotional Support Services

Historically, mental health services have been responsible for directly oppressing LGB people. Homosexuality was classified by the World Health Organization as a mental health disorder until 1992. Most studies about LGB populations focused on the aetiology of homosexuality in the context of mental disorders, with LGB people socially defined within medical terms as 'mentally ill'. As a result, health professionals were often charged with the task of 'curing' LGB people from their 'disorder', using interventions such as electric shock or aversion therapy and starting from the position that heterosexuality is the only acceptable form of sexual expression (Schneider and Levin, 1999).

A textbook on homosexuality and the mental health professions published by the US Committee on Human Sexuality (2000) draws attention to the problem of anti-homosexual bias in psychiatry and psychotherapy, with assumptions that the presenting disorder (e.g. depression) must be a consequence of the client's sexual orientation. This is confirmed by the first systematic study in the UK on attitudes and practices of psychoanalysts and psychotherapists in relation to their LGB clients, which found that clients and patients do encounter overt or covert bias, including the pathologising of homosexuality (Bartlett *et al.,* 2001).

Access to substance abuse counselling services is an important area for LGB health. Substance abuse counsellors hold considerable power and influence over their clients and their attitudes may significantly affect a client's chances of recovery (Eliason, 2000). However, many substance abuse counsellors have very little formal training about the needs of LGB clients and may therefore adopt a treatment approach that assumes that sexual orientation rather than addiction is the problem (Eliason, 2000).

3.6 LGB People and Other Health Care Settings

There has been an increasing recognition within some health care disciplines that the specific care needs of LGB people as service users have gone largely unrecognised (Albarran and Salmon, 2000). In its policy statement on human sexuality, the UK Family Planning Association (2002) summarises evidence about LGB perceptions of the health services and concludes that health services routinely fail to meet the needs of LGB people.

Consequently, many LGB people feel excluded from mainstream sexual and reproductive health services and unable to access what they see as adequate, comprehensive, relevant and appropriate information tailored to their specific needs, such as screening for STIs, cervical cancer and HIV, and sexual health counselling (Fitzpatrick *et al.,* 1994). Knowledge of sexual orientation is particularly important in gynaecological care (Smith *et al.,* 1985).

Other services that have been found to present issues in terms of disclosure of LGB sexual identity and other sexuality-related concerns for LGB clients include accident and emergency (Becknell, 1994), oncology (Mullineaux and French, 1996; Palmer, 1996), midwifery and maternity (Stewart, 1999; Wilton, 1996 and 1999).

Critical care services such as coronary care or intensive care are significant areas because people accessing these services are critically ill, often to the point of life-threatening conditions. Many LGB people will require the services of critical care nursing staff or they will come into contact with these staff because a partner, family member or close friend is receiving care. Albarran and Salmon (2000) reviewed five well-established critical care nursing journals covering the period from 1988 to 1998 and found that issues relating to LGB people are virtually invisible in this field of practice. Studies and debates in this field do not address the needs or concerns of LGB clients and their implications for service providers in critical care settings. The authors argue that this absence will potentially inhibit nurses from establishing effective and caring relationships with LGB patients and from identifying and developing appropriate interventions for the care of these patients and their families. Several other critical care nursing studies have highlighted how clinical staff overtly or covertly convey a preference to care for certain types of patients while others became 'less favoured' (Holyoake, 1999).

Health promotion can also be a problematic area for LGB people where generic health promotion interventions, education programmes and information are underlined by heterosexist assumptions and do not address LGB issues. The Scottish LGBT survey found that between 22% and 28% of respondents had experienced problems accessing appropriate health information (Pringle, 2003).

3.7 Role of Health Personnel

Most authors stress the significance of the role of the service provider in promoting or detracting from the well-being of an LGB person accessing their service. Klitzman and Greenberg (2002) argue that LGB sexual identity may be missed entirely unless clinicians learn how to be open and sensitive to the needs of LGB clients. It is the responsibility of health care institutions and professionals to address homophobia and to create supportive environments in order to facilitate the 'coming out' process in health care settings (Brotman *et al.,* 2002). Health professionals must thoroughly explore their own disciplinary roots and the dynamics of marginalisation and social exclusion that play such a key role in health inequalities (Hall, 1999).

There have been calls for more sensitivity training and the enhancement of homophobia awareness and knowledge of LGB health issues among health system staff in many countries (Yom, 1999; Risdon *et al.,* 2000). It is increasingly recognised that the curricula of medical, public health, nursing, mental health and other allied health professional schools need to do more to incorporate LGB health issues, especially facts about LGB health relevant to their specialisation, and communication with LGB people in general (Ponticelli, 1998). Yom (1999) argues that appropriately trained health care professionals have the potential to improve a society struggling with its prejudices.

3.8 Health Systems and LGB Staff

The issue of homosexuality among health professionals themselves is also a matter of debate. Physicians who disclose that they are LGB to colleagues face the potential loss of referrals and privileges (Yom, 1999; Mathews *et al.,* 1986). Gay or lesbian medical students and residents experience significant challenges and added pressures during their training and their daily work (Riordan, 2004).

The UK Gay Men's Sex Survey found that, in terms of frequency of discrimination, after verbal or physical aggression from strangers in public, the next most common site of aggression and discrimination was in the workplace (Hickson *et al.,* 2003). Studies in North America and Britain report that LGB doctors and medical students encounter homophobic behaviour from both professional colleagues and from patients (Hughes, 2004; Rose, 1994; Risdon *et al.,* 2000). However, others trace the growing acceptance of LGB visibility in the medical profession over the past two decades and claim that the situation of LGB health professionals within the health system has improved even after disclosure of sexual orientation (Yom, 1999).

3.9 Conclusion

The relationship that exists between service users and health service providers is of paramount importance in determining perceptions and experiences of the quality of health care. The level of trust at the interface between the LGB client and the health service provider significantly influences issues of both access and outcome for LGB people.

The question of disclosure of LGB sexual identity features strongly in the international literature as a key issue that has major ramifications for the effectiveness of the patient and health care provider relationship. Sensitivity to the disclosed or potential LGB sexuality of clients among health service providers is essential to overcoming the negative impact of heterosexism in the health system and addressing inequalities in health care for LGB people. The research also points to the problems that are caused by the lack of recognition of LGB familial and social support networks within health organisations and health care settings. These can cause additional stress for LGB people who are already sick or in need of medical assistance.

Research examining the experience of heterosexism and homophobia of LGB people within primary and other health care settings reveals the historical pathologisation of LGB people by the mental health establishment. Two key concerns are the position that service providers take in enabling or obstructing access to health care, and discrimination against LGB staff within health systems.

4

BEING LESBIAN, GAY OR BISEXUAL
IN THE NORTH WEST

The literature review in Chapter 3 highlighted the key issues that impact upon the experiences of LGB people when accessing health care services. This chapter examines what the interviews in the present research tell us about the broad experience of living as a lesbian, gay or bisexual person in the north west of Ireland. The issues discussed include levels of comfort with LGB sexuality, the 'coming out' process, disclosure of LGB sexual identity to others, dealing with heterosexism and homophobia, and the use of support networks.

4.1 Level of Comfort with LGB Sexual Identity

When asked how they felt about being lesbian or gay, all respondents gave a variety of quite positive responses overall, some of which are listed in Table 4.1.

Table 4.1: How Participants Felt about Their LGB Sexual Identity

Gay men	Lesbians
"Love it"	"Okay now"
"Okay, but isolated"	"No problems"
"Grand now"	"Happy"
"Happy enough"	"Comfortable enough"
"Comfortable"	"It is a gift"
"Grand, no choice"	"Makes deep sense"
"Confident"	"Happy and free"
"Integral part of me"	"Liberated"

Many respondents were very confident and comfortable about their sexuality.

"I absolutely love it! It's just me. It's part of my personality. I wouldn't change" (Gay man)

"It's like saying how do I feel about the fact that I am a woman I think, or how do I feel about the fact that I like cooking" (Lesbian)

"I always say I have two gifts in life. One is that I am a woman and the other is that I am a lesbian" (Lesbian)

However, two men and one woman stated that they would rather be heterosexual if they could have a choice, because that would make life easier.

"If I had a choice I wouldn't really want to be [gay], but then, there's nothing gay people can do, you know" (Gay man)

"I have [internalised] homophobia, a large, large amount of it. I don't want to be gay. I'd be much happier to be a straight, ordinary, everyday woman fitting into society" (Lesbian)

One woman described how her feelings about her sexuality could still vary from time to time.

"There are times when … I would have more fear and [worry about] what would happen to me if somebody found out" (Lesbian)

4.2 The 'Coming Out' Process

While no-one gave a totally negative response when asked how they feel about their LGB sexual identity in the here and now, many did refer to the profound difficulties they had in accepting their sexual orientation in the past, for both internal and external reasons.

"If you asked me probably a year and a half ago whether I would prefer to be straight or gay, I would have said straight. But now I will definitely say gay" (Gay man)

For some, the main difficulty was in acknowledging the reality of their sexual identity.

"Accepting it and admitting it to myself was the most difficult part, you know. That took me to the depths and back" (Gay man)

These difficulties were in large part due to homophobia without and within.

"The brother wouldn't talk about it [my LGB sexual identity]. He would give me the look … of dirt and filth. One night, in particular, if there had been a rope in the house I wouldn't be alive today" (Gay man)

"Hugely negative phobia, taboo. Phobias about homosexuality and in every area of life. There was a lot to uncover and deal with over the years, and there was internalised homophobia for myself which I have worked on" (Lesbian)

For others, it was the lack of positive reflection/mirroring.

"There was absolutely no such thing as a lesbian in any kind of visible way" (Lesbian)

Many referred to the lack of support available during the 'coming out' phase.

"I felt there was no backup, there was nobody really to talk to about the situation" (Gay man)

"I thought I was the only one in the world feeling trapped. I thought I was going crazy" (Lesbian)

As a result, some felt the need to go abroad in order to 'come out' (four women and one man declared that they did so for this reason).

4.3 Disclosure of LGB Sexual Identity

Respondents varied widely in the degree to which they had disclosed information about their LGB sexual identity to others, including their families (see Appendix, Table A4). All participants had disclosed their sexuality to at least some of their friends and most (35 out of the 43) were 'out' to all their friends. Twenty-five participants said that they were 'out' to their whole family, while six had not disclosed to any family members. Twenty described themselves as totally 'out' at work or college, while ten had not disclosed their LGB sexual identity to anyone in this context. Generally, participants were glad that they had disclosed information about their LGB sexuality to selected others.

"It [telling friends] has made me stronger ... I feel good about it" (Lesbian)

"... steps like 'coming out' at work earlier on when I started in the job. So being in my work environment, being a place that I didn't have to hide who I was, was quite big and significant" (Lesbian)

There are many factors which governed whether the interviewees disclosed their sexuality to others, including comfort with the issue and the perception of its relevance and safety at any particular time.

"I would describe myself as comfortable, yeah. At the same time, I don't feel I have to go out and tell the world. Maybe years ago I did feel I had to go out and quantify who I was and why I was. But now I've moved on from all of that ... It depends on the context and the setting you know" (Gay man)

"I think the only time when I don't 'come out' is if it's completely irrelevant or if it's detrimental in terms of safety or something like that" (Lesbian)

Some participants chose not to 'come out' at work for fear of losing their job or experiencing discrimination that would in some way impact upon their ability to perform their work functions effectively – five women and two men stated this clearly during their interview.

"I wouldn't necessarily want students or clients to know ... I don't know what they might feel but I am not taking the chance of it impacting on my business and my livelihood" (Lesbian)

Once the process has begun, however, respondents generally 'came out' publicly more and more over time, although the process was acknowledged to be an everlasting one.

"I feel I am always 'coming out' to people, it's an ongoing process. You know at work or whatever, rather than just coming in and saying, 'Well I am lesbian. Now everybody knows'" (Lesbian)

Women participants appeared to be more likely to be 'out' to their families and friends than men.

Bisexual people can feel even more 'closeted' than lesbians and gay men, especially if they are married.

"Married bisexuals fall between two stools ... they are not gay, they are not straight. They don't conform to either expectations ... They would be completely closeted" (Gay man)

4.4 Reactions to Disclosure of LGB Sexual Identity

The reactions of close family members, especially of parents, were very important to most participants when they disclosed information about their LGB sexual orientation. It often influenced their decision to disclose their sexuality more widely or not.

On the whole, reactions from family, friends and work/college colleagues tended to be more positive than negative (see Table 4.2), especially after a common initial period of shock or denial.

"It's been absolutely fine ... and it's been really important to me to be 'out' to those people [immediate family] because I want them to know who I am. They're important people in my life. I don't want to be lying to them about anything. So, it's been a very positive experience for me" (Lesbian)

Responses from immediate family were described as varying from "brilliant" to [they] "think it's disgusting". In a few cases, respondents were asked by family members not to disclose their sexuality to one or other parent for fear of the consequent reaction. This could be difficult for the person trying to come to terms with their identity.

"The only person close to me that I am not 'out' to is my father and that is not my decision, even though it should be my decision. But my mother, for whatever reason, has asked me not to go down that road, at least not yet. It does bug me, it does worry me. But I have to respect that part of the situation" (Gay man)

Some families reacted in a very negative, unsupportive manner to the disclosure of LGB sexual identity by a family member although attitudes may change over time.

"They don't like it, think it's disgusting, not human. That's their opinion on it. Family do not mention it" (Gay man)

"To say the least it was a disaster, [I had a] very bad reaction from the family. I wouldn't say it's even resolved to this day fully. Pretty bad, but it has come around 360 [degrees] since. But it had a huge effect on me at the time" (Gay man)

With regard to friends and work colleagues, most reactions were generally positive after perhaps some initial difficulties. Many commented on their experiences of losing, or potentially losing, previously good friends.

"Eventually, I had to sit her [my best friend] down and say 'This is the situation', and she was shocked. She found it very, very difficult. It took us two or three days of crying and talking about it, and that's it ... no problem" (Lesbian)

"There were one or two people I had spoken with about it [my sexual identity] in [my home town], but you know ... the friendship was severed [as a result]" (Lesbian)

"I mean you'd certainly have a good relationship with some people. There's always the danger that that could be destroyed if a person knew" (Gay man)

Table 4.2: Some Responses to Disclosure of LGB Sexual Identity

Family	Friends/neighbours	Work
"Brilliant", "Perfect" [2 men, 1 woman]	"Fantastic", "Very positive reaction" [2 men, 1 woman]	Fine", "No problems" [4 men, 4 women]
"Fine", "No problem" [4 men, 3 women]	"No problem" [3 men, 6 women]	"Got a little teasing" [1 woman]
"Not spoken about" [1 man, 1 woman]	"Some initial problems" [3 women]	"Regret telling them" [1 man]
"Very bad reaction", "Perverse", "Unsupportive" [2 men, 2 women]	"Lost some friends" [2 women]	

The expectations of the interviewees in terms of a positive response were not very high and many were apparently satisfied with a somewhat qualified reaction.

"You would hear the odd snide comment [at work] but it's water off a duck's back at this stage" (Gay man)

"I have only had one who was my best friend, you know, [she] just slagged me, 'I don't want to mix with you. Oh my God, everybody else will think I am gay'. But no, no ... I have never had bad reactions about it" (Lesbian)

"The main thing is that my family are okay with it. My sisters are all fine. They like know in their own way that it's better for me to be able to identify as being gay than kind of keep it into myself, being in the closet, and sort of having false relationships with girls ... They're not happy about it but they accept it and they're fine with it" (Gay man)

Some interviewees developed a habit of 'sussing out' acquaintances before making a decision to disclose their sexuality.

"Mostly it [the reaction to disclosure of sexual identity] has been really good. But I think that's because I take my time ... to try and figure out how this is going to be with this person. You know, so, I mean I am cautious" (Lesbian)

"I have to know the person I'm speaking to is gay, or sympathetic to gay people. I have to have that background information" (Gay man)

Some interviewees adopted particular approaches to professionals and the public in order to attempt to fit in by restricting the public expression of their sexual identity.

"I think I've probably made a decision that unless it's really crucial I probably wouldn't say ... that I'm living with a female partner or something like that. I think that's the way I restrict myself in terms of what I feel is safe. That's where ... I think it's kind of a modus operandi I have in general to safeguard my own dignity, let's say, in case that I'd be treated worse as a result of telling somebody" (Lesbian)

"We [my partner and I] don't hide it but we don't stand up on the table and announce it either" (Lesbian)

"We know people know, but we just don't wave a flag about it ... you won't see me mincing down [the local town] or walking through [the local town] holding hands" (Gay man)

4.5 Heterosexism

Participants in the study were not specifically asked about heterosexism and homophobia in their lives generally, but during the course of the interviews most made reference to their broad experiences of living as lesbians and gay men in wider society. As outlined in Chapter 1, heterosexism is a widely held set of attitudes and social structures built on the assumption that heterosexuality is the only normal and valid sexual orientation. This in turn gives rise to homophobia – the fear and hatred of gay men and lesbians, which, like heterosexism, can be expressed at an individual and an institutional level. Both phenomena can have a direct negative impact on the lives of lesbians and gay men through ensuing invisibility, exclusion, stigmatisation and even physical endangerment.

Taken as a whole, the comments of interviewees indicate that LGB people in the north west, as with their counterparts elsewhere, experience a wide range of condemnatory and discriminatory practices in their everyday lives. This is already evident from the reports of interviewees about the reactions of family, friends, work colleagues or others to their disclosure of their sexual identity.

Many interviewees discussed how they constantly have to deal with an assumption of 'straightness', whereby people usually operate on the basis that everyone is heterosexual.

"There is a predominant assumption that people are heterosexual ... nobody, whether they're heterosexual or not, gets asked about sexual orientation so that creates the climate of a predominant heterosexual assumption" (Lesbian)

"It's like anywhere in society. People expect you to be 'straight' until you say otherwise. And it's the same in the hospital environment or the health boards. So it's just people's attitudes in general" (Lesbian)

"I live in a tiny little village and everyone is assuming that you are the norm [namely, heterosexual]" (Lesbian)

Respondents stated that anyone who deviates from the norm of heterosexuality is often seen as a 'pervert', or a 'freak', or 'unnatural'. One interviewee mentioned that she had previously lost a job because of her sexual identity; another described an occasion where she received poorer service from a (non-health) professional following disclosure of her sexuality.

Due to the widespread assumption of heterosexuality, many interviewees expressed feelings of invisibility and of isolation as lesbians and gays in the north west region.

"It sounds weird, it's like as if I am asexual for the whole time that I am away from the [lesbian] group … because nobody asks me anything about it … it's not something that people care about, you know" (Lesbian)

"When you're a patient in a hospital or a GP surgery and you're watching TV or listening to programmes or you're reading, there's nothing there on gay matters. There's nothing within the context of communication or in the context of the media within that setting, that says, 'We're open to being gay'" (Gay man)

"It could be a lot easier if I was living in Dublin where there's other gay clubs and pubs. It's more social, whereas in a small town like [my local town] it's not as easy to meet up with other people that are gay" (Gay man)

At the same time, some interviewees reported that, following disclosure of their LGB sexual orientation, their identity is then often seen only in that context.

"When I was in third year [in college], there'd be smart remarks from the first years, 'Ah, there's the lesbian!'" (Lesbian)

A few of the interviewees commented on the legal anomalies that still exist for LGB people in Ireland.

"I should have the same rights. And you don't quite have that. You can't go in and have things like tax benefits etc. etc., because you are a gay couple" (Gay man)

4.6 Homophobia

One female and six male participants described instances where they had heard offensive remarks or were subjected to public name-calling in relation to their sexuality.

"There are instances of homophobia in Sligo … actually quite a number of instances of homophobia and quite aggressive homophobia in Sligo over the last five or six years. You only have to walk around Sligo to see homophobia written on the walls" (Gay man)

"Absolute abuse was coming around the room, before it even got to me. The first things that they thought of when they heard 'gay' was, 'dirty cunts', 'bastards', 'disgusting', 'unnatural'" (Lesbian, recounting her experience of a training course in her locality)

"I found it very hurtful at times what people have said. The fact that they heard someone was gay and what should be done with them. It's very hard to sit and listen to that sort of thing … I've heard a man in particular once saying what should be done with gay people. Of course, what it was, was to be murdered" (Gay man)

One man reported that he had twice been physically assaulted in homophobic attacks, and several others referred to known occasions when such attacks happened to others. Many, particularly male respondents, observed that living in rural areas raised greater fears of condemnation and possible assault.

"I went in to [my local village] at the start, myself and my ex-partner. We expected the tyres to be slashed. I remember when I told my younger sister, she said, 'No problem. Go to Dublin. Don't live here'. [But] I am from here, if I want to be 'out' I will be 'out'" (Gay man)

Women participants were more likely to fear verbal assaults.

"It's present somewhere in the back of your mind. I wouldn't expect to experience physical torment or abuse because of it ... you know, it's all through the side of your mouth that the damage is done" (Lesbian)

One woman described how a publicised assault on a gay man in the local area affected her and her partner. She also alluded to having previously lost her job because of her sexuality.

"I suppose the kind of homophobia that was aired at the time, even in the staff room and all of that, was very difficult to deal with ... I wasn't 'out' there because I was a temporary teacher in the direct employ of the Catholic Church. I had already been ousted from a job which I felt was got to do with the fact that I was a lesbian. Certainly, over the [serious assault on a local man] we were horrified ... That was a very difficult time. That was, I suppose, our realisation here in the west of Ireland that gays and lesbians could be targets" (Lesbian)

Several interviewees alluded to their internalisation of negative attitudes towards LGB sexual identity, whereby the lesbian or gay person takes on and reflects the homophobic responses of society in general. This can lead to denial of one's LGB sexuality in the initial phase and an ongoing aversion to disclosure in certain circumstances.

"I found it [my LGB identity] extremely difficult to deal with, obviously because of my own upbringing ... I thought lesbianism was wrong. I just had to deal with that issue myself and know that it wasn't wrong" (Lesbian)

"I would say there are occasions where I experience internalised homophobia, which also stops me 'coming out' ... It tends to be situations where I'm vulnerable, where I'm more conscious of feeling some kind of ... discomfort about who I am" (Lesbian)

Some interviewees were pessimistic about the prospect of this situation improving.

"The possibility of you not experiencing some form of homophobia is gone, unless everybody accepts the fact that this is natural and normal. And the likelihood of that happening in this lifetime is slim" (Gay man)

Many participants, however, acknowledged that attitudes to lesbians and gays have improved over the years, but that the rate of change has been slow.

4.7 Effects and Coping Strategies

Heterosexism and homophobia led many LGB people in this study to adopt strategies to 'keep out of harm's way', to remain hidden and to avoid disclosing their sexual identity in a cavalier fashion. Attempting to control disclosure is, in fact, a recurring theme in the transcripts.

"You would lie comprehensively to cover it [LGB identity] if need be ... It's a society issue, because as long as people feel they are going to be judged, parodied or ridiculed by society, then they are going to be circumspective of what information they give to society" (Gay man)

"Maybe the way I feel is coming from the fact I was so good at it, so good at hiding how I felt" (Lesbian)

"[I feel] very sad and rejected. It [homophobia] reinforces the idea in your mind that there's no way I can tell anybody that I'm gay. It just wouldn't be accepted" (Gay man)

Despite the fact that most of the interviewees were 'out' to at least some acquaintances, very many commented on their constant vigilance with regard to disclosure of their sexual identity – their sensitivity around who knows and who does not, their desire not to 'flaunt' their sexuality, their fear of rejection and other negative consequences, and their need to get a 'sense' of the person who may be in receipt of the information.

"Some people I won't see any more, but they ask me pretty private questions which I don't like, so they don't get straight answers, just chatting away and at the end they don't know anything about me … They [my friends] would get the right answers. It depends on the sense of what people I can trust" (Lesbian)

A further recurring theme, particularly among male respondents, was the isolation ensuing from social invisibility and reluctance to disclose their sexual identity.

"I feel okay. I can cope with it, do you understand, and face up to it. But, it's the loneliness and isolation that you can't be 'out' … it's a lonely life being a gay person" (Gay man)

Most were also aware of the psychological and physical toll exacted by this constant vigilance, fear, isolation, abuse and internalised homophobia.

"I think the fact of living with discrimination on the grounds of being lesbian, gay or bisexual has an impact on health and has a psychological effect on people and I think that needs to be taken account of … I know people if they even open their mouth they'd get thrown out of the house at the age of 16 or 17. It's a hostile environment for many people … I think it is very difficult and there's huge issues around self-esteem that have to be dealt with in order to successfully 'come out'" (Lesbian)

Most interviewees (21 women and 18 men) have either experienced mental health difficulties themselves or refer to such difficulties for lesbians and gays with regard to their LGB sexual identity. Fourteen mentioned homosexuality as probably being a major factor in relation to suicide.

"It [homophobia] has taken its toll and we haven't actually realised what its toll has been. It has huge effects socially because lots of people move out of the area, go to Dublin and big centres because they can't cope with it" (Lesbian)

Some interviewees highlighted the need for self-protection, often by concealing aspects of themselves relating to sexuality.

"An elderly gay man once in [the local town] – he's dead now actually. He committed suicide, do you know what I mean? I suppose that was why he did [it] too. At the end of the day, he mustn't have been able to cope. I felt it was words of wisdom he told me once when I met him, that – I'm probably talking about 20 years ago or 15 at least – he told me in very strong words, he was very persuasive, to never ever tell anybody you're gay. I felt this was words of wisdom … I suppose he meant that there could be serious consequences from doing so. I suppose what I'm trying to say is perhaps I took his advice" (Gay man)

"Then I come back to live in [my local county] and realise that I slowly start to tuck myself away and tuck bits of me away because of the prevailing attitudes around, not that I have experienced – I haven't experienced – any homophobia. But I suppose I am taking care that I don't" (Lesbian)

4.8 LGB Community Organisations

"I have become more aware of how every day, be it explicit or subtle homophobia, I absorb that and internalise it. And I suppose the best way to contrast it is when I am in a space that is a lesbian space, that is safe – if that's the word to use – but normal. Then I have a whole different sense of relaxation and fulfilment than if I am in the broader society" (Lesbian)

Given the recruitment methodology employed in the present study, it is not surprising that all interviewees professed to be aware of at least some community support organisations, either in the region or elsewhere in the country. All knew other lesbian/gay people living in their localities and most had some lesbian/gay friends. When asked about their involvement in the LGB community, about three-quarters of both women and men claimed to be involved at least socially. Many commented on the role of the community in providing refuge from wider society, especially during the 'coming out' phase.

"[I am involved in the LGB community] because I know what it was like coming through my teens and my twenties having questions in my head and not knowing where to go … and how that can warp a person's development and confidence and self-worth and self-image and all of that … It's about not wanting other people to have the same experiences as myself" (Gay man)

"I wouldn't be maybe as reliant on the gay and lesbian community as maybe when I first 'came out' … It was very, very important for me when I 'came out' that I was able to go out and socialise and meet other lesbians and be in different lesbian spaces that were very, very 'out' and mainly in Dublin. That was really important" (Lesbian)

Most interviewees referred to the LGB support organisations set up in the region – North West Lesbian Line, OutWest, Women Out And About – although men in particular referred to the lack of opportunities for contact with other gay men locally. Consequently, more men than women recounted that they regularly travelled outside the region to attend gay events.

4.9 Conclusion

This chapter presented an overview of what life is like for LGB people living in the north west. All interviewees appeared to be somewhat positive with their LGB identity. However, everyone had experienced heterosexism in their life. There was a general consensus that the reality of everyday life for LGB people in the north west is circumscribed by the challenge of living in a region where there is an assumption that everybody is heterosexual. This pervading assumption resulted in the concealment of LGB sexual identity, the curtailment of behaviour and/or the sense of living an invisible existence for some participants. Feelings of isolation are particularly pronounced for the men who participated in the research.

Self-protection and vigilance are recurring themes with many participants highlighting the consequent psychological and physical toll exacted by constant self-regulatory behaviour. Almost all interviewees associated their mental health difficulties or those of friends and acquaintances with issues relating to LGB sexual identity. Furthermore, 14 interviewees mentioned the likelihood of LGB sexual orientation as a major factor in relation to suicide. Seven research participants had been subjected to explicit homophobic verbal assaults in public, one had experienced physical attack and a number of others lived with the fear of physical assaults.

The experience of interviewees is more positive in relation to the most significant relationships that they have with friends, family and work colleagues. All of the participants had 'come out' to some of their friends, over four-fifths of them had disclosed their sexuality to at least some family members and just under three-quarters had discussed their LGB status with at least some of their work colleagues. In addition, three-quarters of the respondents are socially active in the LGB community and all of them know other LGB people living in the area.

5

FACTORS AFFECTING DISCLOSURE OF LGB SEXUAL IDENTITY TO HEALTH CARE PROVIDERS

Deciding whether to tell practitioners about their LGB sexual orientation emerged as a major concern for most research participants in their interactions with health services. Indeed, it was central to all other themes arising in the study and was found to have consequences for the ensuing health care of LGB clients.

This chapter focuses on the main factors that appear to influence LGB clients when deciding whether or not to disclose their sexual orientation to health care providers. These factors are derived from an analysis of the testimony of interviewees in the study. The opening section, outlining the rate of disclosure of LGB sexual orientation across the services, is followed by an introduction to the main considerations governing the decision of LGB clients to inform or not inform health practitioners about their sexual orientation. The remainder of the chapter is dedicated to a full exploration of each of these factors in turn.

5.1 Incidence

Of the 43 participants interviewed, 12 had never informed any health care service about their sexual identity, at any stage; 22 had disclosed their sexual orientation to some of their health care providers and had not disclosed to others; and nine reported that they regularly disclosed their LGB sexual identity to all health care providers (see Appendix, Table A5).

There was a wide variation between services in terms of the incidence of disclosure of sexual identity. All participants who had attended GUM clinics, albeit mostly outside of the region, disclosed their sexual orientation to the practitioner treating them. Most who had dealt with the mental health services (excluding GPs) disclosed their sexual identity to the counsellor/therapist or psychiatrist, and particularly to private practitioners (see Appendix, Table A6). Similarly, most who had attended complementary health services informed the practitioner about their sexual orientation (14 out of 21 interviewees). Just over half of the participants (12 women and 11 men) disclosed their sexual identity to the GP or practice nurse at some point during the study period, meaning that just under half had never done so. Only one of the 13 interviewees who had spent time in an acute hospital (inside or outside the region) overtly disclosed her sexual orientation to hospital staff. Similarly, very few respondents informed staff in acute hospital services such as emergency and outpatients departments about their sexual orientation.

5.2 Factors

The primary influencing factor identified by participants was relevance: whether they considered disclosure of their sexual identity relevant to their interaction with a particular health service. A number of secondary factors affecting the decision of LGB clients to disclose or not disclose their sexual identity also emerged. The most prominent of these was the perceived confidentiality of the health setting. Other related factors include how they felt about their sexual orientation, their expectations of how the practitioner would respond to the disclosure, the nature of the ongoing relationship between the client and the practitioner and probing by the practitioner in relation to sexual orientation.

"I think you have to tell them the truth when your life is in their hands" (Gay man)

"I've never had any need to 'out' myself. Going to the doctor or GP, there was just a flu, there was no reason to tell them I am lesbian" (Lesbian)

"What determines whether you 'come out' to the GP? I think it's where you are yourself, number one. Then, in the context of the GP themselves, I think it depends on how you feel you can trust somebody, the area of confidentiality, the area that they care about you as a person and not just the physical disease" (Lesbian)

5.3 Relevance to Consultation

The relevance of LGB sexuality to the health care setting may be directly linked with the health condition itself or with some associated aspect that is often linked to relationships. With regards to the former, respondents highlighted sexual/gynaecological health and mental/emotional health as areas where sexual identity is particularly relevant. Consequently, they were more likely to inform primary care or specialist providers in those services about their sexual orientation.

"I suppose something like having to go to the GUM clinic [is where I would disclose my sexual identity] – somewhere where you have to be honest about your sexual orientation. But unless it was necessary I wouldn't feel the need to" (Gay man)

The sexual health issues that prompted disclosure of sexual identity primarily involved thrush infections for women and HIV testing/STIs for men. In these situations LGB clients were aware that their sexual behaviour might well have been relevant to their ailment and was likely to come up in discussion with the practitioner.

"My sexuality is most relevant to me if I have any sexual problems, genital problems. Like, for example, the issue of thrush was an issue for me that I related to my sexual activity. So therefore, it was important for me to say [to the GP] that I was gay" (Lesbian)

In many cases the mental health/emotional issues that led to disclosure of sexual identity related directly to some aspect of the interviewee's sexual orientation and often to a difficulty in recognising or accepting that sexual identity, whether by the client themselves or by their family.

"Literally the minute I walked in the room to her [psychologist] I told her that I was gay … I described myself, as I'm sure loads of gay people do, as square pegs fitting into round holes. Living at home, working at home, trying to have this secret life" (Gay man)

On the other hand, when attending services where sexual identity was not considered to be in any way relevant (e.g. hospital services such as X-ray and outpatients) participants were far less likely to disclose it.

Whether or not sexual identity is directly related to a health condition, however, disclosure may become a relevant issue in any aspect of health care where a person's partner needs to become involved. For instance, where interviewees or their partners were hospitalised for any reason, issues of disclosure typically arose in respect of identifying next of kin, of visitors received, of family involvement in discussions with hospital personnel and so on. In other health care settings too, including primary care, a partner often needed to be involved where any significant decisions have to be made. One interviewee, reflecting on her experience of dealing with health care providers on behalf of her ill partner, highlighted the complexity of the issues involved in disclosing LGB sexual identity, both for clients and practitioners.

"It plays around with who has control over whom you 'come out' to. It's a difficult one. The person who's ill as well has to be considered. There are things about their choices as well. I think it's very complicated … I don't think it's as simple as freeing up staff to be aware of [LGB] identity and to pose that question [to ask a client about their sexual identity]" (Lesbian)

For lesbians these two aspects – relevance of sexual orientation to the health care needed and partner involvement – importantly came together in respect of pregnancy and childbirth (these issues are discussed more thoroughly in Chapter 7).

"For example, if I was pregnant … the expectation [from health care providers] would be, 'Well, where's the Daddy?' and if there wasn't a Daddy, well then they would probably assume that there wasn't anybody. And then if your [same-sex] partner arrives … would they treat the lesbian partner with the same regards as a father?" (Lesbian)

Some LGB clients seemed to ensure that their sexual identity did not become relevant in interactions with certain practitioners by going to a provider or service elsewhere, particularly for treatment on sexual health matters (primarily men, see Chapter 9), or by setting up alternative systems of support with complementary practitioners to whom they felt more comfortable disclosing information about their sexual identity (primarily women). These respondents appear to have designed for themselves a system of health care that allows them to disclose their sexual orientation in circumstances where they deem it necessary or appropriate, and at the same time to avoid the revelation of their sexual identity to their regular or local health care providers. Concerns regarding confidentiality appear to have played a big part in this regard (see Section 5.4).

"I might as well tell you out straight this minute that I'd go elsewhere [for sexual health treatment]. I just could not tell him, for fear, do you know" (Gay man, who during the study period did attend a GP outside the region for treatment on a sexual health matter)

"You see maybe I just have that space with somebody else. Like, maybe I have it with my homeopath, and I have it with my psychotherapist, and I have it with my chiropractor. So I don't need it with the doctor" (Lesbian)

5.4 Concerns about Confidentiality

Confidentiality arose as a major theme for interviewees with regard to the health services generally and concerns around confidentiality inhibited disclosure of LGB sexual identity in some instances. Almost one-fifth of interviewees identified a lack of trust in the confidentiality of the health setting as a primary reason for avoiding the local health services, or indeed avoiding services altogether. This appeared to be the case especially in relation to sexual health, hospitalisation and the work context of some interviewees who were employed by the health services. This lack of confidence was magnified in rural areas where staff may be known to interviewees outside of the health care setting.

"You are going to avoid being tested [for STIs locally] because, you know, Ireland is still a small nation. Everybody knows everybody else, and that is the bottom line. Fear of everybody, that you know information will get out" (Gay man)

"There is always this thing in the back of my mind – I just don't know what people are thinking of me, what attitudes they have … Say I was up in [local hospital], who knows me up there? And who is talking about me up there? … You always expect that confidentiality would be upheld but I don't really think that it is, not in a hospital situation" (Lesbian)

"It would [concern me if I were to 'come out' to my GP] what he would be thinking himself and the fear that he might tell his wife and what she would think as well, because I knew her personally for such a long time" (Gay man)

There were concerns that confidentiality was not guaranteed when using health services. This concern may result in non-disclosure of sexual orientation and, indeed, in non-disclosure of other relevant health data. One man, who himself would "have filtered information" to health care providers because he did not trust that the information would remain confidential, referred to others he knew who did likewise.

"I know of guys who would have withheld information purely because they didn't want people [health care providers and others] to know [about their sexual identity]. And dangerously so" (Gay man)

Sometimes the individual had to prioritise her/his health care needs over worries about confidentiality.

"Each service isn't ring-fenced information-wise. There's a lot of chitter-chatter between people behind the scenes. It's human nature, but I would have difficulty with issues of confidentiality within … but if I needed to go to an STD clinic or something, I would not hesitate" (Gay man)

Sometimes the concern was for children or parents, or not to inadvertently disclose the sexual orientation of a partner.

"Last year I saw the man a lot because I had a really bad ear infection. And I think I didn't 'come out' to him because my partner had been to him before, years ago. And she was shy about going back to him. So there was something about me minding that space or something" (Lesbian)

Others commented that the nature of health care settings is such that they are often not conducive to a sense of privacy and relaxation and that they usually lack any recognition of sexual diversity.

"Sitting in a [GP] waiting room with six or seven other people in and out, you can hear what goes on, who is in there ahead of you" (Lesbian)

"I was thinking when I was talking to … the health nurse … the door was closed over but it wasn't closed. That's just coming to me now. But, probably where I would talk to her about gay issues, I would probably lower my voice, you know" (Gay man)

Those interviewees who stated that they trusted the GP to be confidential with information had usually already informed their health care provider about their sexual identity. In some cases, that trust had developed prior to the disclosure and in others it arose from the GP's response to the disclosure.

"I knew a lot of other students as well who went to her [nurse] and I never heard anything back from what they had been about. When I went in she never discussed anything else about anyone else. So, it didn't come in. I never even thought about it, to tell you the truth. I just knew she wouldn't" (Lesbian)

5.5 Attitude of LGB Client to Disclosure of Sexual Identity

Some interviewees stated that there is no onus on LGB people to disclose their sexual identity at any stage of their interaction with the health services. They asserted that, at all times, LGB people are entitled to make a considered judgement – relating to safety and privacy among other things – on whether to disclose or not, and that a decision not to disclose should not necessarily be seen as a failure on their behalf.

"They [GPs] are there to look after your health as far as I am concerned, and I don't see why gay has to come into it, really … I mean you don't have a straight person going into the doctor telling their doctor they are straight. I don't see the point why I should have to go into a doctor and tell him I am gay" (Gay man)

Some suggested that the main requirement is for the health service to be open to and accepting of LGB sexual identity rather than for LGB people to expose themselves to a possibly vulnerable situation.

"A GP should be able to respond to somebody whether they are actually very confident about their sexuality, or feeling very vulnerable, that they should be still providing an open, accepting service. You know, if somebody doesn't want to open up at that time, well, that's that person's right to do that. But the service should still be open in relation to sexual orientation" (Lesbian)

Others, perhaps more confident in their own sexual identity, have made a deliberate, generalised decision not to disclose their sexual identity to any professional in order to remain "safe".

"I think I've probably made a decision that unless it's really crucial I probably wouldn't say … that I'm living with a female partner or something like that … I think it's kind of a modus operandi I have in general to safeguard my own dignity, let's say, in case that I'd be treated worse as a result of telling somebody" (Lesbian)

From this point of view, disclosure of LGB sexual identity within a health setting is essentially seen as a fluid process responsive to many factors, with any decisions to disclose or not resting ultimately with the client.

"I really believe that as a gay woman we tell people when we're ready" (Lesbian)

5.6 How LGB Client Feels about Her/His Sexual Identity

It appears that the more comfortable the interviewee was with her/his sexual identity, then the easier it was to disclose it to the health care provider.

"It's not that I 'come out' myself [to the GP] and it's not through questions. It's just in conversation. If we're talking about my life, how I talk about it is that it's quite clear that I am a lesbian, more than me actually saying it. Where if they do ask, I do say, 'Yeah, I am'" (Lesbian, who disclosed to most health care providers)

For those participants who were not yet 'out of the closet' in a general sense, it can be particularly hard to disclose information about LGB sexual orientation.

"I'm not used to saying anyway, 'I'm gay' – you know, 'coming out' to people. I've never done that" (Gay man, who has never disclosed to his GP)

A number of interviewees reported that when they were less confident or less open about their sexuality in the past they were less inclined to inform their GP about it.

"It's a pity I didn't have that years ago actually. That I hadn't that opportunity of being comfortable with a GP when I really needed some help, when I was struggling with coming to terms with my sexuality. It would have been lovely to have gone to your doctor and said, 'God, am I going nuts here?' or 'Can you advise me?'" (Gay man, who has now disclosed to his GP)

Others explained how the impetus to disclose to the health care provider came from a need within themselves.

"I just wanted to get it off my chest. I just wanted to get it out because there is no point in having anything boiling inside. Because you become angry, like, you become frustrated. And that's why you want to tell him [the GP, about sexuality]" (Gay man)

A few interviewees suggested, furthermore, that the more confident one feels about one's own sexual identity, the more likely one is to receive a positive response from others.

"I mean the more people accept themselves, I think the more [other] people accept them …" (Gay man)

5.7 Anticipated Reaction of Service Provider

Interviewees were more inclined to disclose information on their sexual orientation when they felt comfortable with the health care provider. However, if the client felt that the reaction of the health care provider was likely to be a negative one, then they were less inclined to disclose their sexual orientation.

(What determines whether you 'come out' to a health practitioner?) "In the context of the GP, I think it depends on how you feel you can trust somebody, the area of confidentiality, the area that they care about you as a person and not just the physical disease ... The other thing is ... their own attitudes and beliefs around homosexuality themselves. Because if they're biased in any way it's not going to be conducive" (Gay man)

"Sometimes, things are acceptable if they're not spoken about, but once they're spoken about, they're not [any longer acceptable]" (Lesbian)

Some indicated how the vulnerability of the patient–service provider scenario is enough to contend with, without the added burden of worrying about a negative reaction to the disclosure of their LGB sexual orientation.

"The more vulnerable I feel in terms of physical or mental health, the less likely I am to 'come out'. I think I talked about when I'm having a general anaesthetic and I know I'm going to be unconscious, I would be scared about being 'out' in case they take the piss or prod you or do something because they know you're a lesbian" (Lesbian)

A few participants identified a very specific fear that may inhibit them disclosing their LGB sexual orientation to the health care provider, namely a concern that the provider will associate their LGB sexuality with some other health-related issue such as depression, child abuse or sexual violence.

"That's always been my fear, is that if I'm 'out' as a lesbian and it's on my records, that I'll be pathologised ... [so if] I'm diagnosed as having clinical depression, that GP's own homophobia will say things like, 'Well, that's because you're a lesbian'" (Lesbian)

"I suppose that fear is there for me, that someone is going to presume that because I was [sexually] abused, that that's why I am lesbian" (Lesbian)

Sometimes the fear of a negative reaction was ascribed to internalised homophobia whereby the LGB client holds possibly exaggerated fears of a negative response. This fear can sometimes inhibit clients from providing useful information to the service provider.

"I didn't want to have to tell her [GP] that I was in a relationship with a woman, that was the main thing. Because I thought that she'd think, 'Well, they're lesbians, they think they're men, they're dead rough'. I suppose I was being pretty homophobic because I was thinking she's going to make assumptions about me – coming in here with this complaint [sexual violence] and I'm a lesbian – I didn't want her stereotyping me or my problem" (Lesbian)

In effect, interviewees where possible often "sussed out" the health care provider before making a decision on whether to disclose their sexual identity.

"I've never had a negative reaction so far from anyone [in the health services] I've 'come out' to – maybe that's because I'm careful about who I 'come out' to" (Lesbian)

5.8 Nature of Relationship between LGB Client and Health Care Provider

The nature of the relationship between the service user and the provider is influenced by the type of health service involved, the health setting and the personality of the provider. For instance, when there is a long-term interaction between client and practitioner, there is a greater likelihood of disclosure of LGB sexual orientation at some stage.

"With my consultant [psychiatrist] and maybe my psychologist, who I'd be seeing on an ongoing basis – [they] would be dealing with me a lot. And I suppose the community nurse as well ... I suppose with them it [sexual orientation] would be relevant, because it's good to have the whole picture. Whereas maybe with nurses as an inpatient in the hospital, it wouldn't be relevant to them" (Lesbian)

The majority of those interviewees who were hospitalised did not overtly disclose their sexual identity to health care providers and some attributed this to the fact that there was little opportunity in acute hospitals to develop relationships with anyone due to the constant turnover of staff dealing with them.

"I was dealing with different people all the time [in the hospital] … There seemed to be no common person I was dealing with … So to 'come out' to somebody there … I was doing it for half an hour and I might never see them again, you know, that kind of thing. So the hospital was just totally different you know [compared with the GP]" (Lesbian)

Infrequent visits to the GP were also cited as a reason for not disclosing information about sexual identity. When clients do not have an opportunity to build up a relationship with a health care provider, they are often less likely to disclose their LGB sexual orientation.

In some instances, the reason for non-disclosure was directly attributed to the manner of the practitioner whereby the client felt that s/he pursued inappropriate or offensive questioning, provided insufficient time for discussion, or was likely to respond in a negative fashion to disclosure of LGB sexual identity.

"I wasn't 'out'. But there were certainly times when, if I had wanted to be, the sort of approach taken by the doctors discouraged me from 'coming out'" (Lesbian)

Some interviewees did not particularly want to develop a relationship with their GP.

"I don't really want a relationship with my doctor, you know, at the same time. I just want to go in and out as quickly as possible and get what I need" (Lesbian)

However, most did wish to establish a rapport, and many referred to the importance of the personality of the provider and her/his ability to put the client at ease. Appropriate listening, questioning and body language gave clues to the LGB client about a possible response, and created an atmosphere of openness and trust which facilitated disclosure.

"If people are friendly with you, you are more likely to disclose information that will probably benefit you and help" (Gay man)

Some participants waited for a relationship to develop over a period of time before they were ready to disclose their sexual orientation to the health care provider.

"I suppose for me the pattern is the relationship building with a doctor, that I am treated as a human being and respected for what my needs are, as opposed to fobbed off. So, I am not going to 'come out' to a doctor the first time I walk in" (Lesbian)

Many participants commented on the often-hurried nature of consultations – particularly with the GP – that discourages an exploration of 'the whole picture'. When a health care provider took time over the consultation, interviewees were more open to disclosing information.

"It was just rushed. I didn't feel at all valued as a woman, not to mind as a lesbian, not to mind as a human being. At least if you had time and whatever and you were taken seriously when you arrive in, you might have some chance of saying it [disclosing sexual orientation]" (Lesbian)

For some, however, the relationship with the health care provider is secondary to other factors.

"I mean the man may have been grand to go and talk to about something, but maybe I wasn't comfortable at the time going regardless of who it was" (Gay man)

5.9 Prompting by Health Care Provider

In some instances health care providers instigated disclosure of sexual orientation by asking pertinent questions, either advertently or inadvertently. Sometimes practitioners directly asked interviewees about sexual orientation and usually received a truthful answer even if the client had not planned to disclose their sexual orientation at that time.

"It was either in the files or she [the GP's co-practitioner] might have been talking to him [the GP] I don't know. But he said to me, 'Are you gay?', and I said, 'I am'" (Gay man)

"I was surprised but I was quite happy that he had [asked about sexual orientation], because at least he was making me feel comfortable and he was making me feel aware that he was aware. Maybe he thought I was holding something back because I hadn't told him or whatever so it was quite a good move professionally from his point of view" (Gay man)

Others, who had not yet disclosed their sexuality to the health care provider, stated that they would respond with candour to a query about their sexual identity.

"If you are registering with the doctor and there is a questionnaire there about your sexuality and yes, I would say, 'I am gay'" (Gay man)

"If the doctor decided for one reason or another, just threw it out on the table to me and said, 'Well, are you [gay]?', I'd say, 'Well, yeah'" (Gay man)

One interviewee, who wished to disclose his sexual orientation to his GP because it was relevant to the consultation, felt unable to broach the subject and needed the health care provider to prompt by asking the relevant question(s).

"I went into him and I said to him, 'I have had a serious family crisis. I am not dealing with it too well'. He probed me a little bit on it, but he didn't ask the right questions … And I felt if he thought it was important enough, he would have asked what was the family crisis" (Gay man)

One interviewee suggested an alternative and less 'in your face' way for health care providers to encourage the LGB client to be more open and trusting.

"It's not necessarily the GP's job to ask people when they come in, 'Are you gay or lesbian?', but it's about having some sort of interaction there, whether it be leaflets in the surgery or posters on the wall or a confidential phone line. That these things are there that people can see when they're sitting in the waiting room or whatever. Because not everybody has the confidence to go in and 'come out'" (Gay man)

Many interviewees have experienced the health care provider making heterosexist assumptions about them, either through behaviour or verbal comments, indicating that they presume the client to be heterosexual. This situation arose most often in relation to sexual health issues and to form-filling. In some cases, the LGB person responded by correcting the assumption and disclosing her/his sexual orientation there and then.

"… all of the doctors I've ever been to have always assumed I'm heterosexual … It just means you have to 'come out' then" (Lesbian)

This was more likely when the relationship already built up between the client and the health care provider was a good one.

"He [GP, on first visit] was dead professional, dead nice and chatting to me. Then, the second time I went in – I think I had thrush. He was just telling me that I should be careful not to pass it on to my partner. He assumed it was a male. Then, I told him I was a lesbian" (Lesbian)

Heterosexist assumptions, however, more often led to discomfort for the client and a reduced possibility of disclosure, either then or in the future. Furthermore, a discomfited client was less likely to disclose other possibly relevant information to the health care provider.

"There was none of them [doctors in GP practice] that I would have felt particularly comfortable talking with about stuff … There was an issue that came up a few months back when I went to see him about something and it was sex-related … He asked me did my girlfriend have the same symptoms. And I said, no she didn't. So that was it" (Gay man)

The following quote highlights the two-sided nature of the whole health care provider–LGB client interaction around this issue.

"I don't think that it's healthy for me to be going to a doctor that's presuming that I am heterosexual. And I don't think it's healthy for me to be going to a doctor that I presume is presuming I am heterosexual" (Lesbian)

5.10 Conclusion

Disclosure of sexual identity, or the question of whether and when it is appropriate to reveal one's LGB sexuality to health care providers, emerged as a central theme of this research. When making a decision about this, respondents took into consideration whether they believed their sexual identity was relevant to the particular health-related issue that they needed addressed and, if so, whether it warranted disclosing their LGB sexual orientation to receive the best treatment. Generally, the evidence outlined here suggests that many LGB service users do inform their providers about their sexual orientation when they deem it necessary for their own health care or the health care of their partners. This arises particularly in relation to mental and sexual health.

However, for a substantial number of LGB clients disclosure of LGB sexual identity is a difficult process and many situations arise where for various reasons they feel the need to avoid disclosing their sexual identity to practitioners. Findings from the present study indicate that an LGB person's capacity to disclose her/his sexual identity to a health care provider may be limited by worries about confidentiality, fear of negative reactions, previous experience of negative reactions and expressed or perceived homophobia or heterosexist assumptions from providers. Those respondents who are less at ease with their sexual identity are less likely to disclose it to their health care providers. Others have learned through life experience that revealing their LGB identity in public may give rise to hostility and disrespect. As a result, they argue that it is generally prudent for LGB people to withhold information about their sexual orientation in any formal context. There are also suggestions from the interviews that other relevant health information may also be withheld from service providers primarily due to concerns regarding confidentiality (this aspect of LGB health will be explored more fully in Chapter 6).

With regard to their decision on whether to disclose their sexual identity, participants often reflected on the nature of their relationship with the service provider – disclosure is more likely in trusting relationships of longer duration – and then made a judgement regarding how the practitioner was likely to respond.

Factors that encourage LGB people to be more open about their sexual identity in health care settings were clearly identified. These included the quality of the relationship with the practitioner and whether the environment: reflected a general openness to the possibility that clients can be lesbian, gay or bisexual; fostered a sense of safety in the encounter in terms of assured confidentiality; and provided a comfortable and private space for consultations to take place. The key issue in relation to these characteristics is not that clients should be expected to disclose their sexual identity but that the conditions are supportive of them disclosing it if they think it relevant and choose to do so.

It is clear that many health care providers are never made aware of their clients' LGB sexual identity and that this can have consequences for the ensuing health care and health-care-seeking behaviour of LGB clients. These issues are explored in more detail in the following chapter, which deals with the experience of LGB clients in disclosing or not disclosing their sexual identity to GP services.

6

EXPERIENCE OF DISCLOSURE OF SEXUAL IDENTITY TO GP SERVICES

Chapter 5 outlined the factors influencing the decision of interviewees on whether to reveal their sexual identity to health care providers in general. This chapter considers in some detail the personal histories of participants when they revealed, or did not reveal, their LGB sexual identity during their specific interactions with GP services. The first section briefly outlines how often and in what contexts respondents were likely to disclose their sexual identity to GP services. Sections 6.2 and 6.3 address the positive and negative reactions respectively of primary care providers to disclosure of LGB sexual identity by clients. Section 6.4 considers the experience of respondents who did not disclose their sexual identity to GPs. The final section explores the consequences, as outlined by interviewees, of disclosing, or not disclosing, LGB sexual orientation to GP services and the implications for many regarding aspects of their health care and health-care-seeking behaviour.

6.1 Incidence of Disclosure

Between them, the 43 interviewees attended a total of 87 GPs and four practice nurses in the north west region during the study period (some interviewees interacted with a number of primary health care providers and some providers were visited by more than one interviewee).

Many participants have never informed any GP about their sexual orientation, some have told some GPs and not others, and some have informed every GP they have encountered. As clients, half of the participants disclosed their sexual identity to just over one-third of the GPs at some point. Twenty-three clients (12 women and 11 men) disclosed their LGB sexual identity to a total of 33 practitioners, including a health practice nurse, during the study period. Of those who 'came out' to their practitioner, most gay men (nine out of 11) disclosed to all of their GPs, while just over half of the lesbians did (seven out of 12).

Most of the 23 interviewees who had disclosed their sexual identity to their GP had done so because they thought it was relevant. The commonest prompts were related to mental/emotional and sexual health issues for both lesbian and gay interviewees (see Appendix, Table A7). In most cases, the mental health/emotional issues leading to disclosure related to some aspect of the interviewee's sexual orientation, and often to a difficulty in accepting that sexual identity. However, this was not always the case, and sometimes the LGB client experiencing mental health/emotional problems simply wanted the GP to 'know' them more.

The sexual health issues that prompted disclosure to GPs primarily involved thrush infections for women and HIV testing for men. Other prompts for disclosure included pregnancy, prescription of contraceptives, transgender issues, and in two cases a direct query from the doctor with regard to the sexual orientation of the client.

6.2 Positive Reactions of GPs

In the majority of cases where interviewees informed practitioners of their LGB sexual orientation (26 out of 33 instances), the GP was described by the client as responding in a positive manner. The characteristics of positive reactions include some or all of the following:

- Relaxed demeanour and body language.
- Reassurance of both acceptance and confidentiality.
- Provision of time and space for subsequent discussion.
- Follow-up queries with regard to supports and health care.
- Provision of tailored information relevant to lesbians, gays and bisexuals.
- No pathologising of homosexuality.

Many interviewees approvingly described how their doctor did not "bat an eyelid" after disclosure, and carried on with the consultation as though nothing had changed. This helped the participants feel more at ease with the service provider.

"He could actually be put forward as some kind of model of good practice – he's never been judgemental, he's never been intrusive and he's never come up with any moral crap" (Lesbian)

"… his response was fine. He didn't bat an eyelid. He didn't care. You were another patient basically. It didn't matter whether you were purple or yellow" (Gay man)

Several commented positively on how the service provider attempted to reassure them and provide them with relevant information or advice.

"He said, 'I totally support you. I have no problems with it whatsoever. I will do anything that I can do to support you. Good luck to you. I hope it [a proposed pregnancy] goes well'. I actually thought that was just a fantastic response" (Lesbian)

"I would see her as one of my supporters … she would say 'Be careful'. (Around sexual activity?) Yes" (Gay man)

Others expressed appreciation of their GP's efforts to ask relevant follow-up questions.

(How did she react when you 'came out' to her?) "Fine, absolutely. You know, sort of, 'Thank you for telling me. I feel privileged that you could tell me. Do you want to tell me any more about it?' Or, 'Is that stressing you, or is that why you feel run down?' She was using it in that sense. She was just so lovely, it didn't faze her at all" (Gay man)

Some also appreciated that their doctors provided openings to discuss the subject on subsequent visits.

"When I visited the second time, she said, 'How's your partner? How are you?' Just in a very – like asking a straight person who's married … By even acknowledging it and saying it meant a lot without having to go into big detail, you know" (Gay man)

Not everybody who disclosed to the GP necessarily wanted to discuss it in great detail.

"I really had liked his response – that he had just been very jovial and he hadn't asked any intrusive questions or had a problem with it. So then he became my GP" (Lesbian)

"There wasn't a problem. She was very professional about it. She didn't go, 'Hmmmm'. She was happy enough. (Did she chat about it?) We chatted briefly. She didn't pry. She didn't go into details" (Gay man, who volunteered the information to his GP as he wished to have a HIV test)

Some interviewees were grateful that their health carers did not automatically relate their sexuality to mental health or other health difficulties.

"When I 'came out' as gay and I had a lesbian partner, she [health clinic nurse] knew that too, but her attitude never changed towards me. She never formed an opinion of me because it wasn't her job to do. She never blamed: 'You're gay, so obviously you're going to need some counselling because of that'" (Lesbian, who attended the clinic for psychological support)

Others requested and received psychological support from the GP around sexuality.

"He's absolutely, extremely supportive. There were an awful lot of issues … that I found very difficult to deal with and he just helped me sort all of those out, and sort out the fact that it was okay to be gay" (Lesbian)

A number of interviewees acknowledged that GPs do not necessarily have all the relevant answers or information to hand.

"It's not that she [GP] had all the answers or that she knew exactly what to do, but she tried her best. She made sure that I had some ideas before I left her office" (Lesbian)

"He was fine … I don't think he knew [about HIV tests], because I asked him, 'If this does come back negative, you know, what's the story?' … and he said, 'Well, I don't know, I am not used to doing this, you know, but I will check up'" (Gay man)

6.3 Negative Reactions of GPs

Interviewees reported seven experiences of negative reactions from practitioners to their disclosure of LGB sexual identity. Respondents experienced some or all of the following reactions from service providers upon disclosure of sexual orientation:

- Signs of discomfort such as lack of eye contact, rushing the remainder of the consultation, a lack of friendliness.
- Lack of an obvious response of any sort or avoidance of the issue subsequently.
- Automatic association of LGB sexuality with HIV status, STIs or other negative connotations.
- Subsequent over-focus on sexuality issues.
- A reluctance to take sufficiently seriously health issues that may be associated with sexuality, such as relationship difficulties.

In some cases the service provider was described as becoming markedly unfriendly and "abrupt" following disclosure of LGB sexual identity.

"He was dead professional, dead nice and chatting to me. When the lesbian issue came up then, he just ran through the rest of it and pushed me out the door" (Lesbian)

"It was his whole action. [His] mannerisms and everything just totally changed, banging things down and so on" (Gay man)

"He got a bit embarrassed about it. You know, he was blushing. I was explaining to him my symptoms then and he was asking me questions [like] was my partner feeling the same. He was really, really awkward about asking me questions" (Lesbian)

In another case the client perceived that she was not being taken seriously when she disclosed herself as a lesbian to the GP. She later described this experience as "not positive" and not conducive to her opening up further to the practitioner.

"My GP, she knows [that I'm lesbian], but I think it's kind of like, 'Yes, yes, well you're going through a phase or something', and I'm saying, 'Hello! I'm 24 years old, you know, so if it was a phase it would be long gone by now, you know'" (Lesbian)

Another client referred to the lack of appropriate follow-up questioning by the GP.

"They [GPs] possibly could have been a little bit more forthcoming, to say, 'Well, how long is this relationship?' and things like that. But, that wasn't really gotten into. Whereas, for somebody who is married, they say, 'Well, how long have you been married? Where did you meet your thing-me-bob?'" (Lesbian)

Some interviewees described how their GPs were unhelpful when they sought support concerning relationship difficulties. The doctor in these cases did not appear to give sufficient recognition to the expressed concerns of the client about her/his relationship. In effect, the doctors again did not appear to ask the appropriate follow-up questions.

"I felt that she didn't really take it [the recent break up of a relationship] on board as an important or a significant issue, and I would have been feeling very, very low at that stage … I went back out of the surgery feeling dissatisfied, feeling not really listened to or not taken seriously" (Lesbian)

One gay man reported that the GP responded to disclosure of his sexuality by immediately suggesting an HIV test for him and his partner.

"Everything was fine and then all of a sudden when you said you were gay, you know, it was like straightaway you should go for a HIV test. Do you know what I mean? Like surely to God, if someone that's straight goes in and has a monogamous relationship and is with their partner for so long and gets an infection or whatever, surely to God they are not told to go and get a HIV test. I doubt it very much … I have never gone back to him" (Gay man)

A lesbian discovered on her second visit following disclosure of her sexual orientation that her GP had written the word 'lesbian' in large letters across the top of her file. She later described this GP as homophobic.

"When I went back she took out my file as such and written across the top of the page, in big, bold print, capital letters, was 'LESBIAN'. So I didn't feel very good about that … you don't want to be labelled and put into a box and everything else kind of irrelevant. This to me, to some degree, showed she didn't really understand what it might be like coming in to see that" (Lesbian)

6.4 Non-Disclosure of Sexual Identity

Almost half of the participants (12 women and eight men) had not disclosed their LGB sexual identity to any of their primary health care providers in the north west region during the previous ten years. A further seven clients (five women and two men) did not disclose to some of their health care providers. These situations, where LGB clients did not inform the practitioner about their sexual identity, arose during interactions with a total of 58 personnel in the primary health care sector (55 GPs and three nurses). In some cases these interactions consisted of only a single visit to the practitioner in question. In others the client attended the practitioner over an extended period.

Most of those clients that did not disclose to GPs said that the issue of sexual identity had not arisen during their visits to date because the issue was not relevant to the purpose of the visits (by far the commonest reason), there was no reason for it to arise or the doctor had not asked about sexual identity. A number of these participants stated that they would disclose to their GP if sexual orientation became relevant to future visits or if the GP brought up the subject in an appropriate context during a future consultation. Many also stated that they would wish to reveal their sexual identity to their GP.

Given the widespread prevalence of heterosexism and homophobia, it is not surprising that some interviewees stated that they would rather not reveal, if possible, their LGB sexual identity to practitioners for safety reasons. However, some interviewees who had not disclosed their sexual identity also experienced increased stress due to fears and conflicts around the possible side effects of disclosure. They tended to feel they were hiding something from their GP if they did not disclose, and yet had fears concerning confidentiality and possible negative reactions if they did.

"People can assume that their GP has confidentiality but the more people that they have contact with in the health board, professional and non-professional and auxiliary services, the more likelihood it is that some of their medical facts or their sexuality may become common knowledge" (Gay man)

"I have to say in terms of confidentiality what bothers me is that even if you have a brilliant GP, you can't guarantee that he's always going to be there. He could die [or] he could leave. Another GP could come along – what if you've got stuff in your records about your sexuality, where does it go, who gets to see it? I think if it's written down somewhere then you lose control over it" (Lesbian)

In addition, some interviewees choose to ensure that they do not have to 'come out' to their regular GP by going elsewhere for health care, particularly when it relates to their sexual health (see Section 9.1). Some participants, in particular gay men, stated that they would rather seek care elsewhere if a 'gay' health problem (i.e. a problem relating to sexual or mental health) arose for them in the future. Many reasons were proffered for this willingness to travel elsewhere for treatment such as increased confidentiality and better treatment. However, others stated that they would be uncomfortable disclosing to their GP locally. This seems to indicate why sexual identity had not arisen as an issue for them with the GP.

One woman and one man, who have previously attended doctors in the city from which they originated, both stated that they would be likely to return to that city outside the region if they were to require treatment with regard to sexual or emotional matters.

"I would go to her [local GP] if there was something physically wrong, but I don't think I would go to her if it was emotional … I would feel easier saying it ['coming out'] to doctors I met in [large city]. I don't know why that is. Maybe it's just because they come across so many – I don't know, maybe so many more people" (Lesbian)

"… if I thought there was something serious wrong with me in that sense [sexual health], I would probably go to the doctor in [large city]. I don't know why. It's probably confidentiality …" (Gay man)

Many other clients, and in this instance mainly women, attended complementary health practitioners to whom they had disclosed their sexual orientation while they had not disclosed to their GP or mainstream health care provider. Here, there were higher expectations of complementary practitioners in terms of openness and acceptance. It is hinted, though, that these LGB clients would still wish to provide the mainstream health care provider with a fuller picture of themselves.

"I would be inclined to go to alternative medicine anyway. And I would be very 'out' in that situation. And it would seem easier to be 'out' I think in that situation. I would love to see a doctor here … that has some analysis of women's lives and women's issues, and lesbian lives in particular" (Lesbian)

Two other interviewees appeared to have set up different sorts of parallel supports where they felt they could disclose their sexual orientation. One woman attended two different GPs simultaneously and had 'come out' to one and not the other. Another woman 'came out' to the nurse and not to the GP in a clinic she had attended in the past.

"As I say, I didn't really know him [GP]. I went to him if there was something wrong medically, he gave me a prescription and I left. But before I went into him, I'd be talking to the nurse first. After I came out from him, I could go back into the nurse if I needed. So, it was grand" (Lesbian, who confided in the nurse but only attended the doctor for brief consultations)

6.5 Health Care Implications

It is possible to identify certain health care implications for interviewees based on whether they revealed their LGB sexual identity to GP services. For those who did not disclose their sexual orientation, a number of health-related outcomes have already been referred to in Section 6.4:

- A greater sense of safety for some LGB clients regarding sexual identity, and more stress for others.

- Increased dissatisfaction with the health service (possibly more cause than effect of non-disclosure of sexual identity).
- More likelihood of seeking health care elsewhere, including outside the region.
- More caution regarding information provided to the GP.
- A less responsive service from the GP.

"Should anything arise in the future, it would be just a much easier situation than having to start at scratch and explain [my sexual identity to the GP] … there would be sort of a knowledge base there, for her. Maybe there is stuff that she would broach with me – knowing that information – that she wouldn't have bothered doing otherwise. Maybe there are questions she would ask that she wouldn't otherwise ask if she didn't know for sure … so maybe it will improve the actual care that I am getting from her" (Lesbian)

For those who did reveal their sexual orientation to a primary care provider, the possible implications can be broadly grouped under the following aspects of health care and health-care-seeking behaviour:

- How I feel about myself and about the practitioner.
- How I feel about my health needs now and in the future.
- The likelihood of my providing further relevant health information to the GP.
- The likelihood of my returning to the GP for further consultations.
- My access to further information and supports relevant to my health care.

These implications are often dependent on the response of the practitioner to the disclosure of LGB sexual orientation.

◦ *How I feel about myself and about the practitioner*

When the GP responded in a positive manner, interviewees tended to feel more comfortable with themselves and their sexual identity. They also tended to feel more comfortable with the practitioner, and developed a better relationship overall.

"I know I've got him now and it's absolutely wonderful to have that back up" (Gay man)

"It gave me the confidence to sort of feel that these things are okay, do you know, and to get on with life" (Lesbian)

"I feel more relaxed maybe going to her now – more confident, because I know she knows everything. Before there was that little package she didn't know. Now she has the whole jigsaw" (Gay man)

In these cases, interviewees were more likely to recommend the GP to others. Indeed, all participants who expressed satisfaction with their GP's response to disclosure of their sexual orientation were prepared to, or had already, recommended that practitioner to others.

"If somebody came to me, a colleague who was gay or lesbian and really needed to see a doctor, I would certainly recommend her" (Gay man)

On the other hand, when a GP reacted to disclosure of LGB sexual identity in a negative fashion respondents felt upset and uncomfortable as a result.

"… basically I just wasn't impressed, you know, the way I was treated. Because basically I wasn't feeling well, I was really in agony and the last thing you needed was that sort of [reaction]" (Gay man)

They also tended to become less confident in themselves and in the practitioner.

"Her verbal reaction [to disclosure of sexual identity] was, 'Oh, that's fine'. You know, she was okay with the idea. But there was just a sense I got that she really wasn't terribly okay with it … I just came away – maybe it was my own personal self-consciousness about the whole gay issue, or phobia about the whole gay issue – but I came away thinking, 'Maybe she just didn't want to examine me'" (Lesbian)

Some regretted that they had disclosed at all, seeing it as a potential vulnerability, especially in a small community.

"I kind of regretted 'coming out' to her. I kind of felt she wasn't as forward-thinking as I thought she might be. Just the minute I felt the vibe, I thought, 'Oh sugar, I wish I hadn't 'come out' so soon' ... Maybe I myself have not really come to terms with meeting her in the shopping centre, meeting her in the town, knowing that she knows something about me, and feeling a little bit of a vibe. I don't know, I just don't know whether I should have said anything or not" (Lesbian)

This woman went on to describe the response she wanted from the GP.

"Maybe she could have verbally reassured me that she's aware of other lesbians in the town or in the vicinity, that she's come across lesbians before and that it will make no difference to her for how she treats me. If she had reassured me that she's still okay being my GP it would have meant a lot to me. Whereas I didn't get that reassurance and I felt maybe it's not okay any longer attending her" (Lesbian)

◦ *How I feel about my health needs now and in the future*
When GPs reacted positively, interviewees felt more at ease about further health care needs from the GP, especially in relation to sexual identity.

"If I felt there was an issue in my life contributing to my medical health due to sexuality, I'd have no problem meeting her and talking to her about it" (Gay man, who is 'out' to his GP)

"I'm not hiding anything from him. I feel that it's a really positive thing, it says something about him as well. It's just really important to me that I can be 'out' to him and that he's okay with it. It means that I can talk about [my partner] if I need to talk about her ... If I have a child, and he's going to be my child's doctor, he will know that there's no Daddy" (Lesbian)

Having 'come out' to the GP and having received a positive response, some interviewees felt more encouraged and at ease to seek further health care elsewhere.

"Now that I have [a GP that I am comfortable with], I probably will most likely go for a smear and the usual tests" (Lesbian)

On the other hand when GPs reacted negatively, interviewees felt that the significance of what they had imparted to the GP went unheard, and consequently that some aspects of their health needs went unseen.

"She [GP] says, 'Well, to regulate your periods you have to go on the pill'. I said, 'Well I can't, I don't want to go on the pill' ... She goes, 'Why?' I say, 'Well, because first of all I am a lesbian and I don't need to go on the pill'. And she never gave me any alternative way of going about it. I think she was more embarrassed about it than I was" (Lesbian)

Even those who felt confident in their sexuality still articulated an awareness of such potential negativity and a desire to avoid extra and unnecessary stress in these situations.

"If I had to go to the doctor in the morning, whether they are gay-friendly or not, I am assertive enough to assert my right. But I don't want to actually have that conflict. Or I don't want to have to deal with those issues" (Gay man)

Clients had concerns about their future health needs from the GP. This aspect seemed particularly important to many interviewees.

"I am a person who wants to have kids and relatively soon, like in the next two years at least. I would like to be able to go to her – because this is my local area and she is a good doctor – and I would like to be able to say, 'Well, this is how I am going about it, and I don't have a partner, and you know, I would rather you not refer to it [my sexual orientation] like that [in a negative way]'. So I would like to be able to do that" (Lesbian)

○ ***The likelihood of my providing further relevant health information to the GP***
Interviewees were more likely to disclose further information that might be relevant to their health when the GP responded positively.

"… anything I needed to talk about, in a general point of view, or a relationship point of view … I could talk to her" (Lesbian)

In one instance, a lesbian client who experienced physical violence from her partner was initially reluctant to inform her GP of her sexuality for fear that the doctor would be homophobic in her response.

"I didn't want to have to tell her that I was in a relationship with a woman, that was the main thing. Because I thought that she'd think, 'Well, they're lesbians, they think they're men, they're dead rough'" (Lesbian)

In the event, she did disclose to her doctor and, feeling accepted by her, informed her of the details of what had occurred. She received what she considered appropriate support and advice as a result.

"She asked me what happened, and I just explained that, you know, that my partner got a bit out of control and she ended up hurting me. She said that violence is violence, and that you can't put up with this kind of violence, and she suggested that I go and talk to the Guards about getting her removed from the house. She advised me that I should go and get professional help and get counselling so that I wouldn't be holding it all in … I felt safe enough to tell her everything, which was something new for me with doctors" (Lesbian)

In these situations, practitioners were also enabled to ask further relevant questions of clients.

"Then we sort of peeled back the onion, and then she said, 'Well, the fact that you told me you're gay ...' and then I started to talk to her about different events in my life ... it was lovely to be able to talk about it, that she had an interest in triggers that may have caused … me to be stressed" (Gay man)

Following a negative response, however, interviewees were less likely to provide or to seek other, possibly relevant, information.

"If she hadn't acted shocked I would have been able to continue my conversation … my question wasn't answered. And it was something I was very worried about" (Lesbian)

○ ***The likelihood of my returning to the GP for further consultations***
After a positive reaction, interviewees were more likely to return to the GP for further consultations. In almost all cases where the response to disclosure of LGB sexual identity was positive, clients remained if possible with the same GP.

"I mean I have no hesitation in going back to her. I don't know, God forbid, if I had some illness related to sexual health, I'd feel very comfortable with her" (Gay man)

"He is still my GP … I suppose the honesty of me telling him, it made me feel more comfortable with him to a degree" (Gay man)

Clients were unlikely to return to the practitioner following a negative response to disclosure of LGB sexual identity. Indeed, only two interviewees in this situation ever returned for a subsequent consultation, although it is notable also that none informed their GP of their reasons for moving elsewhere for further GP care.

"I didn't feel very good about that [GP's reaction], so I haven't been back there since. And I didn't say anything at the time. And I sort of regret maybe now that I didn't, but I kind of didn't feel in a position to say something" (Lesbian)

"After that incident, I don't know if I would go back to her again or not. Part of me knows that I must go back to her just to say, 'I would have liked to have been looked at'. It was negligent really, because I genuinely went in with a genuine complaint you know. I felt it was negligent" (Lesbian)

Of those who did move elsewhere, most found a new GP within the region, but one now attends a doctor in a town elsewhere.

"… for the reasons of the holistic stuff [the GP practises herbal medicine] and for the reasons that they portray themselves as gay-friendly, and also because it's a female practitioner" (Gay man)

○ *My access to further information and supports relevant to my health care*
Once the good relationship between the interviewee and the GP was maintained following disclosure of LGB sexual identity, practitioners were prompted to provide further relevant support, advice and information to clients.

"... if I would call because of my back she would say, 'Well how are you in general?' And I would know that's an opening question and it allows me to go wherever I want with it" (Gay man)

"… he was certainly very, very supportive and would have got me the helpline number for Dublin Lesbian Line at the time" (Lesbian)

In some other situations, interviewees noted that while the practitioner appeared comfortable with their sexuality, s/he did not have to hand any appropriate contacts or information to offer them.

"He could probably find out about the services that are available for lesbians and gays because I don't think he knows ... I don't think that he doesn't want to, but he just doesn't know" (Lesbian)

Following a negative reaction, however, interviewees were less likely to bring up the subject with the practitioner again, even when it might have been relevant.

"I can't bring it [my sexual identity] back to her even though she is a good doctor. *(Why can't you?)* I just feel that initial time when I did say it, and when I got it [a negative response], it's going to be harder for me to say it back to her again" (Lesbian)

6.6 Conclusion

As has been outlined earlier, there are many factors that influence the decision of an LGB client on whether to disclose her/his sexual orientation to health care providers. The present chapter indicates that the act of revealing this information, at least to GPs, can have implications for the health care of the individual, largely dependent on the reaction of the practitioner to the revelation. The decision not to 'come out' to the GP can, in turn, also have consequences for the health and health care of the LGB client. It is clear, therefore, that the issue of disclosing LGB sexual identity to health practitioners is important in the development of a primary care service, and a health care system in general, that is fully responsive to the needs of all its clients.

Given that all interviewees attended GPs during the study period and that the nature of primary care means that an ongoing relationship between client and practitioner is likely to develop over time, it is noteworthy that the majority of general practice personnel in the present study were never made aware of the sexual identity of their LGB clients. Many participants even found it difficult to reveal their sexual identity to GPs when they considered it relevant to their health care to do so. There were many reasons put forward to explain this phenomenon (see Chapter 5) but it is clear that the issue of disclosing LGB sexual identity often creates much discomfort for participants for a variety of reasons. A reluctance to reveal LGB identities in health care settings can lead to avoidance and postponement of interactions with GP services as well as added expense for the LGB client and the possibility of inadequate or misleading information being provided to the health practitioner.

Participants in this research highlighted the importance for them of the responses of health service professionals to disclosure of their sexual orientation. The sensitivities of LGB clients appear to be heightened in this regard and even quite subtle reactions via body language or verbal cues from health care providers can result in positive or negative experiences for the client. In the event, interviewees described most responses from practitioners as positive ones where they perceived that their LGB sexual identity was accepted as normal and did not appear to affect the practitioner's attitude towards them. As has been highlighted by other studies (e.g. Albarran and Salmon, 2000), trust appears to be a central component in this regard. A positive reaction from a GP increases the trust clients establish both in the relationship with that provider and with regard to future relationships with other health service practitioners. As a result, LGB clients are more likely to feel relaxed during consultations, to provide the GP with more information relevant to their health and to return to the GP for further consultations.

Negative responses from service providers can also have an impact on LGB clients by leading to a delay or avoidance in seeking help, a reluctance to reveal other sensitive information to the practitioner and an increased likelihood of transferring to different services elsewhere. These actions may all have implications for the health status of LGB people and have been documented in earlier studies (e.g. Rose, 1998).

There is evidence of generalised positive health benefits for LGB people when they disclose their sexual orientation to GPs (Brotman et al., 2002). In the present study these benefits include a reduction in anxiety for some LGB clients (when the response from the practitioner is a positive one) and the opportunity thus provided for practitioners to offer relevant and useful information. Furthermore, those clients who do not disclose their LGB identity to primary care personnel tend to be more cautious about information they provide to the practitioner and are more likely to seek health care elsewhere, including outside the region if resources allow, especially when a condition arises where sexual identity may be an issue. These outcomes, together with the finding that many interviewees would prefer to disclose their sexual identity to service providers, suggest that practitioners generally need to be sensitive and responsive to the fact that any of their clients may be lesbian, gay or bisexual whether or not this information is actually disclosed to them during consultations.

RECOGNITION OF PARTNERS AND PARENTHOOD

Many respondents raised concerns about the status of same-sex partners and implications for next of kin in relation to health service provision. Some spoke about their actual experiences in this regard and the issue most commonly raised was the importance of the recognition of same-sex partnerships, especially when an LGB client is hospitalised or wishes to become a parent. This again brings up the topic of disclosing sexual identity since, for partners to be acknowledged and included, the LGB client inevitably has to disclose her/his sexual identity to the pertinent health service. A number of women also raised more general concerns regarding their treatment as lesbians if they decide to have a child in the future.

This chapter outlines the main issues that arose in the interviews relating to recognition of partners and parenthood. It addresses partner/next-of-kin matters across the health services generally, but particularly in relation to hospitalisation. It considers the issue of disclosing LGB sexual identity when it is instigated by the desire to include partners as next of kin and reports the concerns of lesbians regarding their health care during pregnancy.

7.1 Recognition of Same-Sex Partnerships

Sixteen respondents (11 lesbians and five gay men) brought up the topic of their partner/next of kin in relation to acute hospital services. Eight interviewees (seven lesbians and one gay man) discussed it in relation to primary care services, particularly regarding circumstances where serious medical decisions have to be made about their health. Six respondents (all lesbians) raised the subject in relation to maternity services and four (three women and one man) regarding their experience of mental health services.

Respondents highlighted a range of experiences where issues of next of kin and same-sex partnerships were responded to by specific health services. Some described positive experiences where same-sex partners were included and acknowledged during health consultations.

"We both attend the same GP. She is completely supportive of us and there would be no question – it [our LGB sexual identity] just doesn't come into it" (Lesbian)

(Would the psychiatrist ever have talked to him as your partner?) **"Oh he did, yes. He talked to him and then he talked to the two of us …** *(As your partner?)* **Yes, as my partner, yes …** *(And how was that experience?)* **No problems … the psychiatrist was actually excellent" (Gay man)**

One participant described a negative experience where she was refused access to information regarding the health status of her same-sex partner.

"I rang [the psychiatric hospital] because I was concerned. I didn't know where she [my partner] was. I just came home and she wasn't here. I was just wondering, 'Is she okay?' They said, 'We can't disclose that information to you.' I went up [to the hospital] then and the receptionist said, 'Are you a family member?' I said, 'No, she's my partner.' She said, 'I can't let you know. Sorry.' … I thought maybe if I hadn't said I was her partner, maybe she might have been a bit more polite" (Lesbian)

Most of the interviewees who had spent time in hospital, plus all the others who brought up the subject of hospitalisation, identified the need and wish to have their same-sex partners acknowledged and accommodated in the treatment and care process and viewed this as a central aspect of their quality of care.

"I feel if I was admitted to [acute hospital] in the morning and I was asked who was my next of kin, I'd like to think I'd feel comfortable by saying, 'It's [my partner]'. That might sound very minor [to others] but to me that would be a major significant acceptance. Or if I was very ill or terminally ill, in relation to my last months or hours or days or whatever, that my partner would be fully included in that package of care" (Gay man)

"In hospital you don't know what's going to happen and there's a sense of powerlessness ... One of the ways of surviving that is through having support. For me, [my partner] has often been my support person and I've wanted her by my side ... if you don't have that, if you can't 'come out' and your partner suddenly has to become a friend, then that relationship is never given the same importance or significance as a partner. So you can potentially lose out on a lot of emotional support that you need when you're in hospital" (Lesbian)

Others suggested that, in instances of serious illness or in emergency situations, recognition, acknowledgement and inclusion of same-sex partnerships in particular were of vital importance to them.

"If I was rushed into hospital and they said to me, 'Next of kin?' … they would probably mean a brother or sister. But I would just tell them, 'Contact [my partner] at such and such a number', and then he would spread the word to whoever would need to know" (Gay man)

"If I was seriously ill as such, yes, I would ['come out']. *(And why?)* Because then you would want to spend time with your partner" (Lesbian)

However, many also expressed deep concerns about what the response of health care providers would be in this scenario.

"[If] I had cancer … I've no doubt my immediate family next of kin would be informed, but if [my partner] went up, who is my partner for the last nine years – out of concern for my partner, would people divulge that information? Would they recognise that he is my partner, as well as my family? I'm not sure that would happen" (Gay man)

In general, those interviewees who brought up the subject of partner recognition:

- Wish to identify their partners as their next of kin (seven expressed a desire to do so, without having been specifically asked by the interviewer).
- Wish to have their partners informed and involved in decision-making around their health care, especially with regard to serious illness (n=7, ditto).
- Held concerns with regard to the legal status of partners as next of kin especially vis-à-vis the rights of blood families (n=7, ditto).

Interviewees suggested that it would be helpful if health service forms recognised categories of partnerships other than those of marital status, with acknowledgement that they can exist between people of the same sex as well as of the opposite sex.

"There was no tick-box [in the health service form] that would acknowledge me living with my partner, being in a relationship for over two years. There was nothing there" (Lesbian)

Some respondents expressed profound doubts whether partners would be accommodated in health-related circumstances and perceived a systematic bias within the health services owing to legal anomalies currently existing around the rights of same-sex partners.

"I don't know that if I have my partner down [on a form] as next of kin, does that hold any weight if anything happens to me? I don't know. My understanding is that it doesn't" (Lesbian)

"I might be wrong but I understand that legally, you know, your next of kin is related to your family, is your family. So what does a GP – or if you are in hospital or whatever – [do] if the partner is on one side of the bed and my father, as it probably would be, is on the other side and they both want different things? You know, that would be very relevant [to me]" (Lesbian)

7.2 Disclosure of Same-Sex Partnerships

The issue of next of kin is closely bound up with that of disclosure or non-disclosure of sexuality for LGB clients. This appears to be the case mostly in relation to hospitals where heterosexism was described by interviewees as being strongly institutionalised.

"I don't have a reassurance in the back of my mind that it's [same-sex relationships] a welcome scenario from the hospital. You are constantly hit with sort of generic male/female [partnerships] obviously. But I have never seen anything to denote same-sex couples" (Lesbian)

"I mean there's nothing. Walking into [my local hospital], there are no triggers for me as a gay man" (Gay man)

Participants' experiences of disclosure of same-sex partnerships to health care providers were varied – disclosure may occur by degrees, with some participants explicitly stating the nature of their relationship to service providers at the outset, while others may provide some information indicating next of kin but no further detail.

Some experiences of disclosure were described as positive and inclusive while other experiences were negative and excluding. One interviewee, who generally disclosed to health practitioners, did so by clearly identifying her partner.

"If I'm asking for permission [to have my partner present during consultations] I'd always say, 'My partner, I want her with me'" (Lesbian)

She also signed her partner as next of kin, in the expectation of receiving the same treatment from practitioners as other patients. In the event, she did.

"As far as dealing with doctors and nurses and anyone like that is concerned, we sort of feel this is who we are and deal with us ... I really feel I was treated as somebody who was ill and needed to be treated. And my sexual orientation had nothing to do with it – good, bad or indifferent" (Lesbian)

Some others signed their partner as next of kin but did not disclose their sexuality in the process.

One participant described her experience of visiting her partner in a psychiatric hospital having previously disclosed her sexual orientation to some health care providers in that service.

"The section [of the hospital] she was in, you had to knock on the door to let you in. They said, 'Be careful not to be too affectionate because of the other patients' ... I don't think that we should have been treated like 'Don't let the patients see that' as if it was something wrong ... I felt they [psychiatric nurses] were seeing us as though we were doing something wrong" (Lesbian)

Two interviewees modified their behaviour with partners so as not to invoke a possibly negative reaction from other patients. Others mentioned this as a concern.

"I've always been in women's wards and you're very aware that their visitors tend to be boyfriends or husbands as well as family members … I'm very conscious of the potential for homophobia from other people who might identify us as lesbians, or [my partner] coming in and giving me a kiss or something. I feel very conscious of how that is perceived and what people think" (Lesbian)

Another reported that her partner did not visit her in hospital at all in order to avoid any possibility of disclosure of their sexual identity.

One interviewee described in detail the circumstances that arose when her long-term partner became seriously ill and subsequently died. In many ways, her experience encapsulates the multiplicity of considerations that arise for LGB clients and the profound emotional and quality-of-care costs when there are no mechanisms in place to recognise same-sex partnerships. During the course of her partner's illness she did not overtly disclose their relationship to most of the health care providers and found herself caught between the desire to respect her partner's wish for privacy regarding their personal relationship and the desire to act as an effective advocate on her behalf (her partner had signed a blood relation rather than herself as next of kin).

"It's a complicated one, unless the two people had it sussed very clearly beforehand. In fairness, [my partner] and I hadn't, we hadn't talked it all through and maybe that was our not wanting to think of these things. We hadn't it talked through, so I wouldn't have felt that free to [disclose our relationship]" (Lesbian)

She did not feel included nor did she experience adequate sensitivity from health care providers to her position as the patient's partner.

"There was quite a start at one time when I said, 'You know, [named partner] would like me to be here'. It wasn't welcomed, but we carried on anyway" (Lesbian)

She described how she tried to incorporate various "allies" to help her.

"I know a lot of the time I worked through the ward sisters. I realised how important and influential a group it can be. They would say something like, 'I'll mention it to the consultant that you'll be there' … That took quite a bit of nerve, even at that" (Lesbian)

She went on to outline the cumulative effects of this on her ability to support her partner through her illness, and on herself as the primary carer.

"It had a huge effect on me … there's a huge amount of thinking that has to happen that wouldn't have to happen if the [same-sex] relationship was explicit and was honoured … I suppose looking back on it now, it lessened my ability to be an advocate for [my partner], put it like that. I think you don't have a position of strength, you are really there on sufferance" (Lesbian)

Another participant spoke about her recent experience of having a baby before she moved to the north west region. During the process, she felt that she had to identify her relationship with her same-sex partner again and again to the various service providers involved.

"… my partner was with me. And they wouldn't let her do certain things or be in certain places because they thought it was a friend and not my partner. So I had to explain again and again" (Lesbian)

Her obstetrician did not wish to allow her partner to be present for consultations and relented only when the woman disclosed her sexual identity and insisted on her partner being present. She later moved to a different obstetrician partly for this reason. She contrasted the consultant's behaviour with that of a nurse who asked her partner to leave when conducting a heel test on the newborn child, when she explained their relationship to the nurse, there was no further difficulty.

Some participants, who did not overtly disclose their sexual identity to health care providers in acute hospital settings, felt that nurses in particular had become aware of their sexual identity primarily through the presence or behaviour of their partner. None of these claimed that their quality of care was affected as a result and asserted relative contentment with this "unspoken recognition" of the significance of the relationship.

"Most of my friends who came to see me [in hospital] were all girls, and I think she [a nurse] would have been there. She came in at a period where the girl that I was [in a relationship] with was there … and she was holding my hand. You'd just know, you'd know it wasn't just a friendship" (Lesbian)

7.3 Parenthood

Four of the female and two of the male interviewees were parents. Most became parents when living in a heterosexual relationship. Generally, the issue of parenthood did not arise frequently during their interviews, and all considered that the issue of their sexual orientation is not relevant to the health care of their children.

Six lesbians, who expressed a desire to bear children in the future, raised concerns about the inclusion of their partners in the undertaking, as well as voicing a general apprehension regarding the anticipated response of health services. All foresaw that they would want, or need, to disclose their LGB sexuality to health care providers during the pregnancy. All expressed anxieties about how they might be treated by the health services as a result, with one woman recognising the debilitating effect of that very anxiety.

"We are considering having a child and I have concerns about that from a medical point of view because I don't know what doctor to go to. It's a critical time and it's a good time and a scary time and whatever. So we just don't know what to do about that at the minute" (Lesbian)

"Are they [staff in maternity hospital] going to treat me differently because I'm lesbian? … If there was a problem with my baby would it be given the same attention as [a child of] a heterosexual married woman? … I wouldn't know what the answers would be but I think living with that fear is as damaging as actually [those] things happening" (Lesbian)

The anticipated response of the health practitioner, especially the GP, arose as a key concern in relation to lesbian parenting. All of the participants acknowledged that they needed the informed support of their GP in the endeavour, but most had concerns with regard to how the practitioner might respond to the idea of a lesbian having a child. Some anticipated a positive and supportive response from their GP while others anticipated potentially negative and judgemental responses.

(Could you see yourself ever broaching the subject of sexuality?) "Oh yes. Yes, I mean if I had an issue, like, for example if myself and my partner decided we wanted a baby I would certainly go to my doctor and broach it with her and say, 'Well you know, how do I go about this?'" (Lesbian)

"They [heterosexual people] could be fine around your sexuality as long as you keep it in the bedroom type of thing, but when you actually talk about bringing a child into the world, then people's moral and religious and all kinds of other judgements come into it. So, even if you'd known that he [GP] was fine about lesbians, you would never [be sure] that he was fine about a lesbian trying to have a baby" (Lesbian)

One interviewee has already been through the process of donor insemination with a clinic in London and found her local GP to be "absolutely fine" with regard to forms that needed to be signed and tests that needed to be carried out for the clinic. However, all of the other respondents who addressed the issue were fearful either that the GP might not be supportive or might not be aware of the particular issues involved.

"If I came to her and said, 'Listen, I am thinking of having a child. I need to get folic acid and whatever', I have to make sure that she is not automatically thinking that I have a partner who is a guy" (Lesbian)

Interviewees also expressed concerns about potential discriminatory attitudes within the health services, particularly maternity services, towards lesbian parenting. One woman, who has worked within the mainstream health system, asserted that she would probably travel to another region with home birth support so that she might have more control over the birthing experience.

"I'm full of apprehension about the maternity services being offered and whether any judgement [will] come into that. I just don't feel I'll get the respect as an equal woman that everybody else would have ... my concern is that there would be judgement and negativity come in and therefore it would sharpen their standard of care and their attitudes and what they're doing ... I've seen all kinds of stuff done and if the staff don't like you, you will pay for it" (Lesbian)

7.4 Conclusion

Concerns about the recognition of same-sex partners in health services were raised by many participants. They expressed concerns about being entitled to access information on their partner's health, being allowed visiting access and being involved in decision-making with their partner in the case of serious health issues. These anxieties were highlighted in the context of a lack of legal recognition of same-sex relationships.

The experiences of some interviewees underline the complexity of situations where there are serious health issues. The lack of legal recognition of same-sex relationships is problematic for both clients and service providers when legal matters regarding consent are concerned. Notwithstanding this, policymakers and practitioners need to ensure that gay-friendly practices take account of diverse sexual identities in order to prevent discrimination within services, to support positive health gain through the involvement of significant others in the care of LGB clients (APA, 2000) and to enhance the use of social networks that are beneficial to health (Braveman, 2003).

Evidence from this study suggests that worries over disclosure of sexual identity and next-of-kin rights can collide to create additional difficulties for those who are inpatients in hospitals where structurally entrenched heterosexism can render LGB people invisible. At times of sickness and vulnerability, when the best possible treatment and support from health care providers is required, LGB people can be further exposed and forced to make stressful choices over disclosure of their sexual orientation. These substantial emotional burdens over disclosure of sexual identity and next-of-kin rights do not apply to heterosexual people in health care settings and, if the HSE and individual service providers are serious about improving equality of access and treatment for LGB people, these issues require urgent attention.

Respondents included those who had children from previous heterosexual relationships and those who had or wished to have children as part of same-sex relationships. Six interviewees were parents of a dependent child and six others, all women, identified a wish to become parents. These potential mothers outlined concerns about their treatment from service providers, either as lesbian parents or in their exploration of the option of parenthood, and one woman described a clearly negative experience. The increasing visibility of LGB people, the greater incidence of families with same-sex parents and new reproductive technologies are increasing the need for service providers to be aware of and responsive to issues for LGB clients in this area of health care.

8

MENTAL HEALTH

Almost all respondents (a total of 39 out of 43) either attended services for mental health support during the study period or referred to mental health as a central issue in the health care of LGB people. Fourteen mentioned suicide in this regard. This chapter explores the key concerns and experiences of respondents in relation to mental health. The first three sections focus on the experiences of interviewees with mental health services.[13] They outline the main reasons why interviewees attended these services, discuss the responses of mental health professionals and consider the experience of psychiatric hospitalisation. The next three sections focus on particular mental health issues of concern to respondents in their relationships with mental health professionals: isolation and stigmatisation of LGB people, pathologising of LGB sexuality and death by suicide.

8.1 Reasons for Attendance at Mental Health Services

Mental health services were frequently accessed by participants during the study period. Twenty-six participants (12 of 19 men and 14 of 24 women) had attended services seeking emotional/mental health support during the previous ten years and 22 of these had attended mental health professionals other than GPs (see Appendix, Table A8). Many attended more than one of the mental health services and some of the reported experiences relate to both public and private services.[14] Four interviewees (two gay men and two lesbians) also had inpatient hospital treatment for mental health issues during that period. In a small number of cases, interviewees attended mental health service providers outside the north west region. This was often, but not exclusively, for geographical reasons because services were not available locally or because referrals were made by GPs to private practitioners elsewhere.

A variety of factors were identified as the primary reasons for consultations with mental health professionals. The most common overall factor was attributed to depression associated with sexual orientation. Interviewees who visited their GPs when feeling depressed or 'low' at some stage during the study period ascribed their feelings, at least partially, to such factors as discomfort with their sexuality, their family's discomfort with their sexuality, the stresses of 'coming out' or problems in relationships. Many of the key reasons cited for respondents' use of mental health professionals other than GPs were also linked to sexual identity (see Appendix, Table A9).

---

[13] In this study, unless stated otherwise, mental health services are considered in a broad sense to include any emotional or psychiatric/psychological support provided by mental health professionals to LGB research participants during the study period. This includes psychiatrists, counsellors (including rape crisis and addiction counsellors), therapists, psychologists, psychiatric nurses, other staff of psychiatric hospitals, general practitioners, social workers and other specialised support personnel.
[14] Thirteen of the 43 participants had attended a health board psychiatrist during this period, while 14 had seen a private therapist or counsellor.

"When people are very low and they're accessing some of the services from the health board – for example [for] alcoholism – but behind all of that maybe [it's] something to do with their sexuality. When you peel back the onion, just because people access services and it has nothing [overtly] to do with sexuality, you never know indirectly that sexuality might come up. People are very vulnerable in that" (Gay man)

The following quotes illustrate how the experience of heterosexism and homophobia can be a significant factor contributing to mental health problems for LGB people.

"… both from my own experience and talking to and knowing other lesbians, I think the impact of exclusion and homophobia and all of the fears of rejection and of labels of everything from pervert to very unwell, diseased person. That has to have an impact in terms of one's mental and emotional health and spiritual health" (Lesbian)

"As a lesbian … I have all this negative internalised homophobia that I need to address and work through. And that's where it's relevant in psychotherapy and whatever else" (Lesbian)

8.2 Approach and Responses of the Mental Health Professional

Interviewees generally wanted to be heard, accepted and understood by both GPs and mental health professionals, including counsellors, therapists and psychiatrists. Time and time again, participants reiterated this point in many different circumstances. Most interviewees who had experience of the mental health services emphasised the importance of being given the space to simply talk and to feel heard, especially in relation to LGB sexual identity.

"I needed somebody to listen, very much because a lot of the [counselling] process was about hearing myself speak and sorting out through the chaff … a lot of 'coming out' is actually having their ears" (Gay man)

"It was just brilliant. The difference was that there was somebody there to sit down and talk to. Your sexuality wasn't an issue. If you wanted it to be an issue, they sat and they listened" (Gay man)

"I was very depressed at the time and I went and I told him [my GP] I was feeling very, very depressed … I had hoped that he would have probably referred me to someone to talk about it. Sort it out. But he just scribbled out a prescription for anti-depressants and gave it to me" (Gay man)

Another emphasised how having someone to talk to, in this case a health board psychologist, helped him to overcome suicidal feelings in relation to his family's negative response to his sexuality.

"Having talked to him has helped an awful lot, because I felt good. I felt relieved at the time I 'came out' after having talked to him. I felt that he helped me through it" (Gay man)

One woman made the point that being provided by the professional with a space to talk and feel accepted in is even more important than having relevant information to hand.

"If a doctor or a counsellor, especially doctors, if they listen and then they ask questions about what you've just said, then you feel a lot more free to be able to talk to them and be able to tell them exactly who you are and exactly what's on your mind … And it's not even about information they have. It's to do with what kind of person they are" (Lesbian)

Others commented on the cold manner of some practitioners that discouraged engagement.

"When you sat talking to [the psychiatrist], you talked to his ear … he looked off to your left, so you were talking and looking at his ear. So facial expressions [are important]. I didn't see [his face] to judge" (Gay man)

A few interviewees referred to how the physical surroundings contributed to the comfort of the counselling process.

"It's a really caring and safe and comfortable environment they've created up in the Rape Crisis Centre. It's not horrible tables – there's no tables. There are really comfortable seats, cushions all over the place if you want to sit on the ground. There's flowers and plants. *(Does that make a difference?)* Yeah, it's not an office, it's a comfortable room. You feel more homely. You feel comfortable and safe to be in that environment" (Lesbian)

In addition to being heard and accepted, research participants also emphasised the necessity of being understood by mental health professionals. A lesbian experiencing depression through living in a closeted and difficult same-sex relationship, and who was referred to a psychiatrist by her GP, felt that the former did not grasp the issues involved.

"… in terms of my sexuality there was no kind of understanding [from the psychiatrist] of what the issues were. You know, in relation to being in this relationship and being kind of stuck … She didn't, I feel, understand" (Lesbian)

In this case, the psychiatrist proposed what the client considered highly inappropriate solutions, including a stay in a psychiatric hospital and a night out in Dublin.

"… at one stage, she suggested that I go to Dublin and book in somewhere and go off to a lesbian event, a disco or something like that, and go off with somebody else for the night … I don't know what her rationale was behind it, but I just thought, 'I know this is not right for me. I don't know what this woman is talking about or where she is coming from, but I have had enough'" (Lesbian)

Instead, the woman left the psychiatrist and returned to her GP for counselling and he provided her with the telephone number of a lesbian helpline, which she found more useful.

"I might have needed more support. I might have needed more connection with other women, but I think the manner in which that was suggested … I suppose the contrast was, you know, [my GP] giving me the number of the Dublin Lesbian Line. They are very different types of support than just saying, 'You go off now and find somebody for the night'" (Lesbian)

In retrospect, she attributed the attitude of the psychiatrist to a lack of understanding on the whole issue of LGB sexuality.

"I think she sort of had all the [language], you know, 'This is fine' and all that. She had that language initially, but if you were to read through it in how she made that suggestion of me going to Dublin and then being cured, you know, suggests to me that she wasn't actually okay about it. She didn't really have an understanding" (Lesbian)

Very often, it is this "lack of appreciation of what the issues might be" for LGB clients, rather than outright homophobia per se, that participants highlighted in cases where they were not happy with mental health professionals. This was often evidenced by the practitioner ignoring issues associated with LGB sexual identity that may be relevant to the counselling process, or not taking such issues seriously enough. Both situations are illustrated in the personal accounts outlined above.

It is noteworthy that interviewees tended not to inform the professionals of their dissatisfaction with the service provided. Also, apart from the incident described above where a GP provided the interviewee with the number of a lesbian helpline, none of the other interviewees indicated that they sought or received any information from mental health professionals on LGB support organisations.

Another lesbian compared her experience of two health board psychotherapists. The first therapist she found to have little understanding of LGB lives (the therapist was a trainee at the time).

"She was talking about relationships as if there was no difference whatsoever between lesbian relationships and heterosexual relationships – that lesbian relationships emulate heterosexual relationships. I didn't like that, I thought it was a kind of heterosexist assumption or whatever" (Lesbian)

She then requested a transfer to a second psychotherapist whom she perceived to be more helpful and who, unlike the first, managed to separate her sexual orientation from her mental health status.

"She [the second therapist] is not pushing her own heterosexuality down my throat. Again, she seems absolutely cool about me, no problem at all about me being a lesbian and she's very, very good … She's consistently kind and warm and positive and she doesn't pathologise. She doesn't make out [that] my sexuality might be a contributing factor to my mental health" (Lesbian)

She elaborated further on the value for LGB clients of a good counselling technique.

"It means that I don't have to worry about being a lesbian. I don't have to think badly of myself for being a lesbian. I don't have to be ashamed. I don't have to feel guilty. I don't have to link it in with my mental health anymore … It means that I can pay attention to all the other things that I need to pay attention to [in the consultation] rather than trying to hide or dismiss or invalidate my own sexuality … It makes me have more confidence in her as a practitioner" (Lesbian)

A total of six research participants stated that they would have a preference to attend a lesbian or gay (or gay-friendly) counsellor or therapist, but that personnel with these attributes are not available or are not publicised.

"What would be really, really helpful would be a gay-friendly counsellor of some sort, male or female … or, in a perfect world, gay themselves, so that they would have a connection there already and know where you are coming from … So, you're walking in and you know the counsellor gets half of you already, which is good" (Lesbian)

All emphasised, however, that the primary requirement is for an all-round professional who is "sussed" about LGB sexual identity.

"I am not certain there needs to be somebody labelled as being openly gay-friendly or gay themselves or whatever, for support. I think it's more important that there is an understanding that they are open. Period" (Gay man)

8.3 Hospitalisation

Four participants, two lesbians and two gay men, had been hospitalised locally for psychiatric treatment at least once during the study period. Three of them had more than one stay in hospital. Both men stated that their sexuality was linked to their hospitalisation but neither of the women did. Experiences of the hospital environment varied among the four interviewees. One lesbian did not conceal her sexuality while in hospital and reported that she did not experience any overt homophobic behaviour from staff.

"… a few nice long conversations with some of the nurses about it [my LGB sexual identity]. They were fine. They were helpful. They were nice about it" (Lesbian)

The second lesbian, who was not 'out' generally, had a more mixed experience. For example, a nurse passed "smart comments" alluding to her LGB sexuality while in the company of others and sometimes remarks were passed about other gay patients in the hospital. On the whole, she did not consider the hospital to be a gay-friendly environment.

"It happened on a few occasions, yeah. It would be a few, you couldn't say they were all like that, but there would be a few members of staff that wouldn't be too positive about it [LGB sexuality] … I wouldn't like to see somebody going in there now – say for instance, somebody who was having difficulty accepting their sexuality" (Lesbian)

8.4 Isolation and Stigmatisation

Respondents made constant and insistent references to the silence and the perceived lack of support that contribute to a sense of isolation and stress for the individual LGB person in daily life. This also arose with reference to how the mental health issues of LGB clients are perceived by some health services personnel. Interviewees suggested that in situations where they do not feel adequately supported by mental health professionals, for example when issues associated with sexuality are not acknowledged or are not taken seriously enough or are problematised in a negative fashion, then this reinforces the sense of isolation, of non-acceptance and of being misunderstood for the LGB person. There was a widespread perception among interviewees that support is not available from the health services for an adequate understanding of LGB people's mental health.

"I know about people who have experienced physical and mental ill-health because of difficulty accepting their own sexuality … The health services aren't really doing anything about that" (Lesbian)

"There was nobody [in the mental health services] kind of cared less, do you know. And … with the psychiatrist and the hospitals and that, I felt it [my LGB sexuality] just wasn't an issue. But yet to me at that time it was a big issue, you know" (Gay man who, due to difficulties in accepting his LGB sexual identity, had taken an overdose)

"I think there are common threads of being frightened about it [LGB sexuality], being accepted, about getting support, about getting direction, about follow-up. About somebody out there that you can get some counselling with, or advice. That, as far as I'm aware of, doesn't happen" (Gay man)

The sense of isolation is exacerbated by the inherently vulnerable nature of the counselling/ therapeutic situation. One man, while struggling to deal with 'coming out' and the consequent break up of his marriage, attended the emergency department in a local hospital after attempting suicide. There he met a psychiatrist who spoke to him for some minutes and who sent him away with no follow-up appointment.

"I just felt I was at the end of my tether to be quite honest and I took an overdose and then I was brought to accident and emergency. But I spoke to a psychiatrist then and there was absolutely no back-up service whatsoever … if I had known there was somebody, you know, that I could have spoken to … But I mean there was nothing …" (Gay man)

The man later attempted suicide a second time and spent a period in a local psychiatric hospital attending the same psychiatrist.

"When I said to the psychiatrist [for the second time, when in hospital], 'I am gay, my marriage broke up' … he brushed the issue aside, you know. It was kind of 'Get on with it, it's not an issue'. But I suppose at the time it really was [an issue for me]" (Gay man)

Another man had a similar experience of not being 'heard' by mental health professionals in the region.

"Certainly they [health board counsellors] had a total lack of appreciation of the significance and importance of the dwarfed development emotionally and psychologically of a closeted gay person, and how it affects them and how they interact with others … I found that very hurtful and very undermining" (Gay man)

Both these men went on to find what they considered more useful support from private therapists outside the region.

Some interviewees approached mental health professionals with a degree of distrust, especially in the initial stages.

"If you're in a confused or depressed state, particularly for instance like the period when I was in transition, that could be a potentially dangerous time to be involved with the mental health service … I have been treated disrespectfully by males particularly in the mental health services in England. I wouldn't have the same confidence that I would be treated seriously" (Lesbian)

"Before I went [to the counsellor], a few people had said she might be a bit prejudiced towards [me] being a lesbian … I talked to her [counsellor] about my fears, about the fact that she mightn't be comfortable about me being a lesbian. She reassured me that there was no problem with it at all. That it was not even an issue" (Lesbian)

The sense of isolation exacerbated the need to maintain confidentiality and in some cases led to interviewees avoiding local services and travelling to other regions to avail of mental health services. Two interviewees stated that they would not seek help from local GPs if they ever needed emotional support, rather they would return to attend practitioners from their native (large) city outside the region.

"I don't know why that is. Maybe it's just because they come across so many more people … Or you are less likely to see them walking down the street" (Lesbian)

8.5 Pathologising LGB Sexual Identity

Two lesbians described experiences where their LGB sexual orientation was pathologised by mental health professionals, a third respondent used the label in relation to the experience of her partner and a fourth interviewee expressed fears about such an eventuality. In these cases, the clients perceived that practitioners intrinsically linked or might link their lesbian sexual identity with their mental health difficulties in a negative way, while they themselves were clear that it was not an underlying factor for them. For instance, a counsellor suggested to a woman who was dealing with her adoption as a child in traumatic circumstances that her LGB sexuality simply derived from the loss of her birth mother.

"[She said] 'You are not really gay, you are only looking for a mother substitute'" (Lesbian)

Another, who experienced clinical depression on an ongoing basis, feared informing her new GP of this in case he attributed it to her LGB sexual identity (in the event this GP did not fulfil her fears following disclosure).

"I was also concerned that because I had this history of having clinical depression and being prescribed anti-depressants that he would then make a moral judgement or a medical judgement that I wouldn't be fit to be a mother. What I was worried about was that some of his own prejudices about single mothers, lesbian mothers, would come into that, that he would justify it with mental health. He hasn't done that at all … I think it's really boosted my confidence" (Lesbian)

Another interviewee, a survivor of child sexual abuse, was constantly afraid that GPs would automatically associate this with her LGB sexual orientation. She avoided the situation by not disclosing to any of her GPs, even though she is aware that heterosexism and homophobia have impacted on her mental and physical health.

"I have become more aware of how every day, be it explicit or subtle homophobia, how I absorb that and internalise it … in terms of my health, how it impacts is the stress, be that in my immune system being weakened, or being anxious, or getting an odd panic attack, or whatever way that it manifests itself" (Lesbian)

Similarly, a respondent avoided mentioning his sexuality when he sought help from his GP for depression since he did not want her to presume that his gayness caused his mental health condition.

"I came back and just went [to the GP and told her] about feeling a bit down in myself. I didn't discuss being gay or anything like that … I just didn't want her to think that just because I was gay that that's why everything felt a bit black for me at that time" (Gay man)

On the other hand, a lesbian described a positive experience with a psychiatrist who did not automatically pathologise her sexuality and label it as the basis of her mental health problem.

"When he determined that it [LGB sexuality] wasn't the major cause of why I was there [emergency department], he dealt with the cause of why I was there … It made me feel quite calm, because I knew I was being listened to" (Lesbian)

8.6 Suicide

One-third of interviewees (ten gay men and four lesbians) spontaneously brought up the issue of suicide in relation to LGB sexuality. One man had attempted suicide twice and another had seriously considered it in the previous ten years.

"Things weren't going right and I felt wasted and I felt that I should pull the plug if I could. That was really the main big issue – me being gay and the family not accepting it. And I just felt that, well, if I was out of their way they would never have to worry about me. Then one night in particular I would have [attempted suicide] … Several times I thought about it" (Gay man)

Six gay men and three lesbians knew others who had died by suicide (in all cases, male) and attributed it to problems in relation to their sexuality. Participants felt that difficulties with being gay in a homophobic and heterosexist society had contributed to suicidal feelings and the decision by these men to die by suicide.

"The last three funerals I would have been at were [suicide] funerals as well. And I do think it's basically down to, a lot of it's down to sexuality" (Gay man)

"When I was there [in the psychiatric hospital], I met one of the male patients. He was there for a while and he was gay. He was purely in there because he was thrown out of his house and he tried to kill himself because he was gay" (Lesbian)

"It's just I wasn't getting any support at home. I actually attempted suicide as such. But it wasn't suicide, it was a cry for help" (Lesbian, speaking about an experience of more than ten years previously)

Furthermore, it was the perception of these respondents that LGB sexuality is a bigger contributing factor in suicides than is widely recognised and that it needs to be given greater attention if LGB health is to be improved.

"Some of those young men that are committing suicide are gay men. I know them, they come from my own area, you know. Some are actively gay or are known to be gay, but others – who knows? They're just young men who committed suicide and who knows" (Lesbian)

The silence around the issue of sexual orientation in relation to suicide was emphasised.

"And there is no doubt about it, one of my firm beliefs is that young people who are struggling with their sexuality … a lot of it, you know, ends in suicide, which is a tragedy of huge proportion, but it's not talked about, because it cannot be proven. I know one young guy alone who committed suicide who I knew was gay but nobody else or very few others had known" (Gay man)

8.7 Conclusion

A substantial number of participants in this study had experienced emotional distress and/or mental health problems. Apart from problems associated with disclosing sexual identity, the most significant issues that respondents raised in interviews were difficulties relating to mental health, mental well-being and service provision. The majority of interviewees who brought up the issue of mental health linked it to their sexuality. However sexual identity in itself is not a cause of mental health or emotional difficulties. Rather, it has been shown that the link between higher rates of mental health problems and being lesbian, gay or bisexual is due to a lack of acceptance of LGB sexuality, fears about or experience of negative reactions and discrimination due to LGB sexuality (Morris and Rothblum, 1999) and isolation from social support networks that have been shown to be protective of health (Wilkinson and Marmot, 2003).

One-third of participants made a link between emotional distress and suicidal feelings or actual suicide attempts. The issue of suicide and its link with sexuality arose spontaneously in interviews, unprompted by any questions. Several people anecdotally mentioned men they knew who had died by suicide and for whom they believed being gay in a heterosexist/homophobic world was a significant contributing factor. The experience and views of participants reflects international evidence that there is a link between suicide attempts and sexuality, particularly for men (Remafedi *et al.,* 1998).

The experiences of respondents who accessed mental health services because of emotional or psychological distress varied. Many sought support for problems associated with their sexual identity but not all did. Generally, interviewees stressed the need for mental health professionals to offer a welcoming, listening space and to have sensitivity to all the issues involved. Traditional attitudes within psychiatry have pathologised LGB sexual orientation and are still felt to have an impact by reproducing homophobic attitudes within mental health services (Bartlett *et al.,* 2001). In the present study, even supportive service providers were not always felt to have an understanding of the particular experiences of LGB clients and the impact of heterosexism on their lives. There is evidence that some people, due to their sexual identity, travel outside the region to access mental health services elsewhere. The value of supportive and accepting services was clearly identified as important for respondents to achieve acceptance of themselves as lesbian, gay or bisexual and to acquire a positive view of their sexual identity.

9

SEXUAL AND GYNAECOLOGICAL HEALTH

Most of those who participated in the study discussed LGB sexual identity in relation to sexual/gynaecological health and the sexual health services. In the vast majority of cases these issues were raised spontaneously by interviewees rather than in response to questions from the interviewer. Many respondents asserted that sexual orientation was relevant to their sexual health and that LGB clients had specific needs of the health services in relation to sexual and gynaecological health.

This chapter describes the experience of respondents in accessing sexual/gynaecological health services and the key issues that arose in relation to them. It considers the sexual health service provided by GPs and outlines the experiences of participants in genito-urinary medicine (GUM) clinics. Section 9.3 contemplates issues related to gynaecological health and the final section charts the concerns of interviewees regarding the lack of knowledge around sexual/gynaecological health issues, particularly for lesbians.

9.1 Sexual Health and GPs

Sixteen of the 19 men and eleven of the 24 women interviewed raised the subject of sexual health specifically in relation to GPs. Of these, four men and five women attended GPs in the region for consultations regarding sexual health matters during the study period (one man also accompanied a gay friend to a GP in relation to sexual health). Three of the men attended in connection with HIV tests, and three of the women attended for treatment of thrush infections (the remaining conditions were unspecified). Eight of these nine clients disclosed their LGB sexual identity during their consultations, if they had not previously done so. This was usually, but not always, in response to the practitioner making an assumption that the client was heterosexual.

"The first female doctor I went to when I came back [was] because I had thrush, and that was the first time I went to her … I can't remember, you know, what the phrase was. It was basically, was I married or had a partner or whatever. And I said I was lesbian and I said, yes, I had a partner" (Lesbian)

However, one interviewee felt unable to declare his sexual identity to the GP in these circumstances.

"He asked me did my girlfriend have the same symptoms. And I said, no she didn't … I suppose I was uncomfortable to turn around and say, 'Well, it's a fella'. He just assumed straightaway [that I had a girlfriend]" (Gay man)

Three respondents (two men and one woman) mentioned that a GP had asked them about sexual activity in relation to safe practices and in each case the GP was either already aware, or was subsequently made aware, of the sexuality of the client.

"I was in [with my GP] with a particular problem, it wasn't sexually related. He asked me was I engaging in unsafe gay sexual practices or was I operating safe … I was surprised but I was quite happy that he had, because at least he was making me feel comfortable and he was making me feel aware that he was aware [of my sexual identity]. Maybe he thought I was holding something back because I hadn't told him [I was gay] so it was quite a good move professionally from his point of view" (Gay man)

Three of the four men who consulted their GP on sexual health issues also went outside of the region to GUM clinics for routine sexual health tests during the study period. In addition, two other men chose to attend GPs outside the region entirely for treatment in relation to sexual health matters. One man and one woman also stated that they would go elsewhere for treatment if something of a 'personal nature' arose in the future. The main issue for these clients was the desire to avoid having to disclose their sexual orientation to their home GP and a concern regarding confidentiality. All of those who travelled away for sexual health services did so without referrals from their local GP and usually without their knowledge also.

"If I thought there was something serious wrong with me in that [sexual health] sense, I would probably go the doctor in [home city]. I don't know why. It's probably confidentiality and because he knows everything about me so I wouldn't have to go through reams of questions" (Gay man)

One man expressed an awareness that not all LGB people necessarily have the information or contacts to arrange a consultation outside the region and consequently may not be receiving adequate health care.

"Currently the only method of doing it [HIV testing] is either through your GP, through the GUM clinic or going to Dublin. Which … for some people means that it doesn't happen" (Gay man)

Many participants did, however, report satisfaction with the GP's response in relation to sexual health issues and highlighted how, in some cases, the practitioner proceeded to ask relevant questions about sexual practice with a comfortable and non-judgemental demeanour.

"I was so worried sick. I went to my doctor and I explained the whole thing to him and he was fine. I said, 'The doctors up there [in the GUM clinic] could ring you if there was a negative or a positive [result] or whatever. I'm just letting you know'. He said, 'Don't worry. Don't worry. I'll look after you. I'll look after you' … He's a fantastic doctor" (Gay man)

"It was more a sexuality issue, but I felt quite comfortable saying to her what I had to say [about my condition]. She makes it very easy for me to talk about things … I think myself she's more in touch with what's going on for me than any other doctor's been. I feel free maybe to say, 'Look I don't feel very sexually active at the moment', or, 'What's going on for me, is it because of the change of life or what is it?' and she's open to anything I say" (Lesbian)

However, some participants also reported unsatisfactory experiences. One gay man left a GP who had failed to treat a testicular infection following disclosure of his sexual identity, to attend a second practitioner who was "friendly" and prescribed antibiotics. One lesbian tried out two GPs regarding a sexual health matter before she found, on a third occasion, a practitioner who she felt was comfortable with her LGB sexual orientation. Another man expressed concerns that GPs may, on hearing that the client is lesbian, gay or bisexual, have HIV or STI tests undertaken without permission of the client.

"I wanted to be sure that my blood wasn't being tested for things against [my will]. Like I didn't want a HIV test through work and I didn't want a drugs test through work unless it was mandatory and I did explain why. She [GP] said, 'No, we were only testing for this particular hepatitis strain and we need your consent for anything else'" (Gay man)

Another participant felt the GP inappropriately responded to disclosure of LGB sexual identity by immediately raising the subject of HIV.

"I did have an [STI] infection as well. And he said, 'Well maybe you should get her to come in and see me'. So then I explained to him that my partner was a male, and that I was gay. And as soon as I said that he said, 'Oh, oh right', and his attitude changed totally … and then he said, 'Oh well maybe we should send you for screening and maybe we should get you HIV-tested and things like this'. *(Did he make an appointment for you or anything?)* No, no, no, no, no … *(So did you go back to him again?)* No, never, never" (Gay man)

This man later attended another doctor with his partner for an HIV test, but found that the doctor, while helpful, did not offer sufficient support in terms of the test.

"Even the doctor, like he wasn't even aware that you did need someone there for counselling … if the test came back and it said, 'Yes it is positive', that you are HIV-[positive], does the doctor just tell me that and there is no-one there, you know what I mean? … There was not even a leaflet or anything" (Gay man)

9.2 GUM Clinics

Eight male and no female interviewees had attended GUM clinics during the study period. All participants who attended GUM clinics disclosed their sexual orientation to the practitioner treating them. Three had visited clinics for HIV tests, two for general STI checkups, and three gave no specific reason. Six of the eight men went elsewhere to visit a GUM clinic despite the fact that there is a clinic located in the region. The reasons put forward for travelling outside the region were to have more anonymity, to access more specialised medical expertise and because the geographically nearest GUM clinic for some was located outside the region.

"I still think I am in a more anonymous position going to [a large city] than I would be going to [the local GUM clinic] … It's the [local] clinic. I would be worried about" (Gay man)

"The lads, like, my group of friends, would always tell you to go to the sexual health clinic [in a large city] as opposed to the doctor. So I mean, I just feel a lot happier that they [the clinic] deal with it a lot better. They deal with it on a regular basis and the expertise would be a lot better, you know" (Gay man)

The need for anonymity and confidentiality in accessing GUM clinics was raised as an important issue by a number of participants. In two cases it influenced where participants accessed the service. In addition it influenced what specific service respondents consulted – two participants stated that they attended GUM clinics for sexual health checkups in preference to consulting with their GPs for reasons associated with increased anonymity.

Particular confidentiality issues related to concerns about being seen going to the clinic locally and/or meeting service providers that may be known to respondents. Two men commented on the inappropriate location of the local clinic. Both mentioned the lack of privacy in the approach to the clinic as a potentially inhibiting factor for gay men.

"When you live and work in the [local] area, you fear walking into a GUM clinic and be staring face to face with a professional who you know personally. Your boss or a neighbour or a relation or somebody who knows you. And aside from it being a very bloody awkward moment it's a potential nightmare … You can't crack the whip against them and tell them, 'You will not talk'" (Gay man)

Actual interactions with GUM clinic personnel, both locally and elsewhere, were described in a uniformly positive manner with interviewees finding them gay-friendly and non-judgemental as a whole. No-one reported that clinic personnel had made any prior assumptions about their sexual orientation and some described how questions were asked in an open-ended and sensitive fashion. The importance of such an approach in enabling a person to engage with the service was highlighted.

"I met him there [in the local GUM clinic], the Men's Sexual Health Officer. I have to say he was absolutely brilliant at his job. He is so open-minded, friendly … He asked was I gay, heterosexual or whatever, and I told him and he was absolutely brilliant … Now I was iffy about being there for the first time but I mean he made me feel so comfortable. More than that, I suppose I was brushed aside so much prior to that that I really didn't know what to expect" (Gay man)

9.3 Gynaecological Health and GPs

Many lesbian respondents discussed gynaecological health and GPs. Most of the experiences related to cervical smear procedures. Twelve participants stated that they had had a smear test in the previous ten years. In all cases, the practitioner who carried out the procedure was a female GP or female practice nurse. Three interviewees attended GPs for other (unstated) gynaecological conditions during the study period. Of the participants who had had smear tests, half described it as a negative experience. Some of the reasons given, such as the physical pain and discomfort involved, are potentially common to all women, while some are exclusive to lesbians, in particular the impact of assuming that the client is heterosexual. Four women reported that the GP or nurse carrying out the procedure revealed through their questions that they assumed the client to be heterosexual.

"She did this smear test and then I talked to her about the post-menopausal bleeding. In relation to one or the other she asked me if intercourse was painful. That made me really angry – that she assumed I was heterosexual [and] she assumed I was sexually active. She made a lot of assumptions about me without respecting me, I felt, because I did find her questions offensive" (Lesbian)

Three of these participants described having the smear test as a frustrating or upsetting experience, and none revealed their sexuality to the relevant practitioner.

"Then, as she was putting the speculum in, she said something like, 'How long have you and your husband been trying to have a baby?' … I managed to not answer her questions by going, 'Aaoouuw!' or something … I just thought that whatever her intentions were well meaning, health practitioners when they assume you're heterosexual and then it's your job to put them right and you never know how they're going to react. You're in that kind of vulnerable situation and that's happened to me a lot in the past when I've been having smears or internals" (Lesbian)

None of these three participants gave the practitioner any intimation of their distress.

"I didn't [tell the GP that I was upset]. I should have done and I wish I had done, but I didn't. I just told her I wasn't sexually active. I didn't discuss anything with her … it's the only time I've ever seen her, so I don't have a relationship with this doctor. I didn't particularly have any confidence in her as a person to talk to. [There hadn't] been any respect" (Lesbian)

In addition, of those three interviewees, one stated that she provided less information to the practitioner as a result and one commented that she would rather not return to have another smear test carried out.

"Obviously, I need to have regular smear tests and I would be very reluctant to go back to her, very reluctant. I'm the kind of person who would just avoid it" (Lesbian)

One participant highlighted a situation where potentially negative impacts arising from assumptions of heterosexuality were dissipated owing to the response and attention received from the GP.

"I felt that she gave me the care that I wanted, that I wasn't just a number. She sat down with me and she wasn't rushing me out the door or anything. A few months later then the pain came back … she was asking me was intercourse painful for me and I told her then that I was gay and that I wasn't in a relationship at the time and that I wasn't sexually active or anything. That's how it came around. I felt totally at ease saying it to her" (Lesbian)

Eight of the 24 lesbian interviewees acknowledged that they had delayed or avoided having cervical smear tests. Again, some of the reasons given are potentially common to all women. These include earlier negative experiences, not knowing any doctor with whom they'd be comfortable having a test and fear that the test might uncover cervical cancer. However, the other reasons provided for delay or avoidance are exclusive to lesbians. Two respondents felt that, as lesbians, such procedures would be too intrusive.

"They would need some improvement there for the likes of me to go in [for a smear test]. But being gay that would put me off going in there … It's pretty personal" (Lesbian)

"I don't know if they can change the size of these contraptions that are used to keep the vagina open as you are trying to get a smear … If you are not, you know, used to penetration then it might be even more traumatic than someone who is, anyway. But I guess you know there are lots of … single women who would be straight who would be in the same situation" (Lesbian)

Six women suggested that lesbians have less risk of developing cervical cancer than other women, but some professed to be unsure of this. One woman reported incidents with GPs indicating that some health practitioners are no wiser.

"I know I was told in Dublin [by a GP] that I didn't actually need to get a smear test if I was a lesbian … And my first GP that I went to in [my local town], asked me did I need to get a smear test. So she actually asked me, 'Do lesbians need smear tests?'" (Lesbian)

This interviewee claimed that she had not yet taken a smear test partly for this reason. Another respondent alluded to the "naivety" and ignorance of lesbians generally around sexual/ gynaecological health.

"Just because we are lesbian, we tend to overlook those smear tests, I think, generally. We are not as good as a heterosexual woman in doing that … I think we are naive in a lot of cases as you think you cannot contract AIDS because we are lesbians … So I think, just sometimes, we are a bit blasé about the whole thing" (Lesbian)

9.4 Awareness of Sexual and Gynaecological Health

Seven of the 24 women interviewed referred to the lack of knowledge around lesbian sexual/ gynaecological health issues, whether amongst lesbians themselves or amongst health care providers. They emphasised the dearth of information on lesbian sexual health as compared with that available for gay men.

"Well, if a medic asked me if I was sexually active I would say, 'Yes, absolutely'. But the literature I would have ever read around smear tests etc. would have been – I would [have] understood it to be heterosexually sexually active. So that's where I think of going, 'Oh well, that doesn't refer to me', and of course it does" (Lesbian)

Participants commented, in particular, on the absence of lesbian sexual health information in doctors' surgeries.

"I think some of my fears around not knowing what the right thing to do is, as a lesbian, in terms of sexual health and looking after myself … I don't have any book, other than [to] learn from others or talk to people. So I feel like a kind of teenager going into a gynaecologist or a doctor or something and asking them to guide me" (Lesbian)

"In the waiting room there are a lot of leaflets on sexual health. The leaflets that you get now are mainly to do with sexual health for men and gay men … If you don't feel included in some service, you won't go. You might go because you have to, but you won't feel comfortable there and you won't make the most of it" (Lesbian)

In contrast, many of the gay men seemed relatively informed about their sexual health. For instance, very many gay men identified the taking of blood tests as situations where there is a responsibility on gay clients to disclose their sexuality to medical personnel (predominantly in relation to HIV/AIDS protection and blood-related illnesses).

"Me and my friend both went to [GUM clinic outside of the region] back in June just to have an STD checkup done because we thought we needed it. Just to get the first one over and done with, we thought if we went together and got it done, because it's something that you should do pretty regularly if you are sexually active" (Gay man)

Some interviewees suggested that the lesbian community ought to become more proactively involved in sexual health advocacy work and in the development of lesbian sexual health information.

"That's where I'm talking about information for lesbians. I don't know if I have to or I don't have to [have a smear test], or whether I'm less at risk or [at] a higher risk. It would be nice to have that information" (Lesbian)

9.5 Conclusion

Sexual health was identified by a majority of the participants in this study as a key issue for LGB people. Overall, the male respondents were primarily concerned with the provision of gay-friendly sexual health services, while women stressed the need for gynaecological health services that are appropriate for lesbians. Confidentiality was a significant concern in relation to sexual health matters, particularly given the rural nature of the area. Some interviewees said they preferred to access services outside of the area that offer more anonymity and are better geared towards their specific sexual health needs.

The question of travel to services elsewhere, by LGB people who are dissatisfied with or do not feel comfortable with the health care options that are available to them in the north west region, brings up further issues related to equity of access within the health services. Inevitably, some people will have the information and resources that enable them to access alternative services elsewhere and some will not. LGB service users who do not have access to information on the services available elsewhere and how to procure them, or those without sufficient financial resources or access to transport, are not in a position to choose to go elsewhere even if they are unhappy with the service they receive locally as LGB clients. This is particularly an issue in a predominantly rural area like the north west that has a relatively high level of economic disadvantage and a poor transport infrastructure. There are indications from the interviews, moreover, that this inequity may mean that some LGB people may delay, postpone or avoid reporting health conditions to local practitioners, especially when they relate to sexual or mental health.

Some interviewees had unsatisfactory experiences with GPs in relation to sexual/gynaecological health. Often this was because the GP assumed that the client was heterosexual or appeared to be uncomfortable when an LGB client disclosed her/his sexual identity. Again, there were indications that this might lead the client to reveal less information to the practitioner, to seek help elsewhere or to postpone seeking health care altogether. Although the experiences of interviewees with GUM clinics were uniformly positive there was a lack of consistent knowledge and awareness of sexual health issues for the LGB population, particularly with regard to lesbian health. This situation has also been observed elsewhere.

Almost half of the women who participated in the research had not had a cervical smear test and half of the group who had undergone the procedure described it as a negative experience. All the women who had a smear test preferred or requested that a female practitioner conducted the procedure. A positive finding in the research is that all the female participants reported that this need was met by their local health services. Many lesbians had delayed or avoided having smear tests partly due to a widespread and erroneous understanding that lesbians are at less risk of acquiring cervical cancer. Some of the interviewees were critical of the lack of knowledge amongst health care providers and amongst the lesbian population itself concerning the general sexual/gynaecological health of lesbians and the data suggests that doctors and nurses in this field require comprehensive awareness training around the health and service-related needs of their lesbian clients.

10

SUGGESTIONS FOR IMPROVED HEALTH SERVICES FOR LGB CLIENTS

Throughout the interviews participants made many suggestions about how health services could be improved. These suggestions, which were made both in the course of discussing aspects of services and in response to direct questions from the interviewer, represent a set of 'steps in the right direction' to enhance the experience of LGB clients using health services. This chapter draws these suggestions together, grouping in sequence the proposed specific actions for the health system generally, for all health care providers, for particular service settings and finally for LGB people themselves.

10.1 The Organisation

◦ *Emphasise a culture of 'equal rights' rather than 'special treatment'*

"It's not about having separate lesbian clinics or whatever necessarily, but it's about where, you know, from the policy-making level to the cleaners on the floor level, that there's more of a culture change. It all needs to be backed up with very clear statements about not being treated prejudicially" (Lesbian)

Some participants suggested the need for the HSE to develop an organisational mission statement with a reference to LGB people having equal rights to access health care services and to quality of care, within an overall equality and diversity policy. Participants stressed the need to see an explicit organisational commitment to equality for all clients and, in particular, LGB clients.

"I would prefer if I could see statements on the wall, equal opportunities statements and stuff like that. That would make it easier, yeah. It changes the nature of the environment, changes the quality of safety in the environment. Otherwise you don't know what you're walking into" (Lesbian)

"So that, look, despite whatever you might practise or whatever your personal opinion is, that you will treat a patient the same, no matter what race they are, what age they are or what sexuality they are. I guess the knowledge of that somehow portrayed would make it easier" (Lesbian)

◦ *Counter heterosexism and homophobia across the organisation and in all services*

"It is important that with the health providers there is an acknowledgement of homophobia. And there is a challenge of homophobia with practitioners, so there is training for frontline services" (Lesbian)

Participants stressed the importance of acknowledging and challenging heterosexism and homophobia at an organisational level. Such an approach would involve the support of senior management, visible displays of information on LGB health and the introduction of awareness training. It was considered vital that support for these actions emanates from the top levels of the organisation.

"At the end of the day it's about leadership and taking the initiative. We've all these policies. I smile when I think of the health strategy – 'patient- and people-centredness'. Taking that in the context of gay health, there you have a theme within a national context to do something. But that takes strong leadership, strong drive by the CEO. If it's seen that the CEO – I know he can't influence everybody – but if he's bought into it, I think it will ripple in if there's a drive there. It has to be seen from [the] top down and [bottom] up. But nothing will happen unless someone takes leadership around it" (Gay man)

○ *Acknowledge that both patients and staff can be lesbian, gay or bisexual and raise the visibility of LGB people throughout the health service*

"Even having a poster on the wall for straight people to see and understand there are gay people in the community. It might help to get rid of some of the prejudices. Even have the statistics up there … That people would think, 'Well, there's one in every extended family at least' and that it's okay. That's just not realised by [heterosexual] people, that people are living their lives under wraps" (Gay man)

Many participants suggested the need to name and include LGB people on visual material, forms and documentation through all health care settings. They stated that this information would indicate openness to LGB issues within the health service and would send out a positive message of the legitimacy of LGB identity within the wider community.

"There is nothing in there that makes you feel welcome as a gay person. If there is something on the wall about lesbians and gays, you might feel more comfortable going in" (Gay man)

"It is important that the administrative system accommodates for LGB people. If the form says, 'Do you identify as lesbian, homosexual, heterosexual, bisexual?' If it gives me a list of choices that allows me to feel recognised and acknowledged … So I suppose I want the health system to give it visibility. Don't, as a practitioner, reinforce the exclusion" (Lesbian)

○ *Introduce and influence more training on LGB issues and the social context and about specific medical issues for LGB patients*

"We should introduce education and training around LGB issues and explore staff attitudes" (Gay man)

Participants suggested the need to work with all health professionals to develop, deliver and monitor sexual orientation awareness-raising and skills training. This training would include both undergraduate and in-house professional development levels. It would enhance the possibility of heightening sensitivities to LGB issues, thus leading to the development of 'gay-friendly' services.

"In their training generally, it would be nice to know they do a module of work on gay and lesbian issues, that the GPs have to do a study on something on gays and lesbians, that nurses have to do something. So that the general public know that the health board personnel have actually done some module of work on the whole issue of sexuality generally … then they'd have to discuss face to face their own sexuality, plus look at the possibility of other sisters, uncles, aunts [being LGB], you know – just [that there's] more out there" (Lesbian)

"It's hugely important that health [service] people dealing with the public, as part of their training, that there is an appreciation of some form of education as part of their training, on lesbian and gay issues" (Gay man)

◦ *Work in partnership with the LGB community and groups concerned with LGB health*

"I think the act of reaching out to people is hugely important to people who feel marginalised and alienated … it doesn't have to be that everybody is sorted out about everything, but that there's an active sort of engagement with struggling to understand something or to respect something like that and to acknowledge something different" (Lesbian)

Some participants suggested that forming partnerships, engaging with LGB interests, and funding more community supports for LGB people would enhance the experiences of LGB people utilising the health services.

"I think the health board has a responsibility to get involved with gay people, [to] go out and reach gay communities or groups, a bit like the Samaritans. Get yourself out there and know you can contact us or whatever. I think they have to take a huge step in raising awareness that they are open to gay men and women, which may generate a culture then for gay people to use the services. Then it may encourage people who aren't 'out', to avail of the service or to open up" (Gay man)

◦ *Work proactively with the education sector*

"Just like there was some big promotion [on dental health] in schools recently, maybe if there was [a] nationwide campaign every so often, where personalities or some people from the health board gave in-service to teachers and came into schools to talk on the whole area of sexuality. I think that would be huge" (Lesbian)

Participants stressed the importance of working jointly with all levels of the education sector on the design and delivery of programmes to inform about sexual orientation issues and to challenge prejudice and ignorance. In particular, participants highlighted the importance of providing awareness-raising supports for LGB youths. Suggestions proffered in this regard include:

- Organise a programme of workshops on diversity for students, making LGB sexuality visible and acceptable.
- Contribute to training teachers on sensitivity towards LGB issues.
- Produce posters, leaflets and flyers on sexual diversity for distribution to schools.
- Make counselling services available to young people exploring their sexual identity within the school setting.

"I would see the [HSE] having quite a large role to play in educating people, parents and school-going kids of an appropriate age … because it [sexual identity] is just not touched on. But it's such a fundamental part of a person's existence, their sexuality. Being gay or straight is such an important part of them and defining them as people … I feel there's a huge area that's ignored or it's being tackled wrongly in getting information out there to people. It's cutting a potential problem before it ever really becomes a problem" (Gay man)

◦ *Deal with the issue of same-sex partners and next of kin in health care settings*

"I want to have the choice of bringing my partner with me to scans, to exams, to whatever pre-natal stuff is happening and for her to be accepted as my partner, and that there's some acknowledgement that partners [of women] can be women, that partners are not always men" (Lesbian)

Participants identified the need to design and implement ways of improving support for and acknowledging same-sex partners as main emotional supports during treatment and home aftercare and also their role as next of kin.

"Certainly inclusion for a partner in any decisions and consultations [is needed]. I think there's a question, 'Who else would you like?' or if a family next of kin is there then a question may be, 'Who else would you like to be included?' [or] 'Is there anything else that would make it so you that you'd be more supported?' I suppose it does focus on asking what the needs are of the patient, and then including those people who love that person in whatever is to be told or said or consulted about" (Lesbian)

"When taking a [client's] history, because of the way I've put the questions together, I hope that it just encompasses all of everything [that's relevant], which is, 'Is there somebody special in your life and what status do they have?' I would never actually come right out and ask if they were gay. That to me is irrelevant in my work. What is relevant is the relationship they have with their partner – you know, are they happy within it? That's the relevant part, not what sort of relationship is it" (Lesbian, who works in the health sector)

10.2 The Individual Health Care Provider

○ As service providers, seek and secure training about LGB issues and perspectives and about specific medical issues for LGB patients

"You know you expect doctors and people that are working in health issues, that they shouldn't be ignorant. They have been trained. They know per se what a homosexual is. They know it's a genetic thing. They know that it is not a mental disease. I can go back to when I was a teenager. I can understand that ignorance, but not forty years later" (Gay man)

Participants suggested the importance of all health professionals educating themselves about LGB issues and perspectives. This could be achieved through attending professional and/or in-house training programmes around sexual orientation and LGB issues related to health.

○ Do not assume clients are heterosexual, be more respectful and accepting of difference

"They should have that bit more respect for the gay person so that he or she has more confidence in coming to use services, so they can be honest with themselves rather than [having] to hide things and keep it behind closed doors" (Gay man)

Participants highlighted the need for health care providers to demonstrate an open-minded approach to sexual identity, to avoid the assumption of heterosexuality and to maintain an acceptance of difference in their service delivery.

"A gay-friendly service would make me feel more comfortable. It would feel friendlier. I would feel more relaxed because I would know that there wasn't in the first instance a presumption that I was heterosexual. So that sort of clears the air for you and levels the ground" (Lesbian)

"The health professionals have an obligation to not make assumptions about somebody's sexuality. For example, if women are having smears, you don't ask a question, 'When was the last time you had sexual intercourse?', because there is an assumption that you have sexual intercourse. If health professionals work out exactly what information they do need in order to carry out the procedure and then find a question that can elicit that information that isn't making an assumption. I think there's ways and means of doing it" (Lesbian)

○ If an LGB client decides to disclose her/his sexual identity, react appropriately

"I won't know [how the service provider is going to react] until I tell him. But a good reaction would be a start. A professional reaction would be great – hopefully [it would] be expected. I would hope he would have some checklist, or some type of way of dealing with the gay community" (Gay man)

Participants highlighted the importance of proactive reassurances from the health care provider on disclosure of sexual identity. In particular, participants suggested:

• Health care providers should be aware that disclosure is often difficult for clients.
• Reassurances are essential pre- or post-disclosure, namely that the health care provider is familiar with the issue, has dealt with the issue before and/or is comfortable with the issue.
• Be ready to give time to the client as s/he might want to talk about the issue further.
• Use questioning techniques that leave opportunities for the issue to arise and that do not assume heterosexuality.
• Do not make automatic associations between LGB sexual identity and health conditions such as HIV, child abuse, mental ill-health and so on.

"What would make me more comfortable is if they didn't have the presumption that I was straight, number one, by asking some kind of question that indicated I am straight without knowing. Then, if I did tell them [that I'm lesbian, that] they wouldn't have a problem with it" (Lesbian)

"I would want that they [service providers] are comfortable dealing with you. And that if you are going for blood tests, that they [do] not assume he has AIDS right away. And if you are going for that test, that you've a fear that you're [wishing to be] well received and that you're not treated like a leper and that you're still human and you're coming for things to be done the same as a straight person" (Gay man)

◦ Be sensitive to what stage an LGB client is at in the process of 'coming out'

"There's an issue for yourself, how 'out' or not you are, [that] has a huge bearing on how people are. I understand people getting annoyed, 'How was I supposed to know?', 'How could I assume?'" (Lesbian)

Participants outlined the complexity of the 'coming out' process for clients and stressed the importance for health care providers to be sensitive to what stage the LGB client is at in this process. They suggested the need to look for subtle clues and to ask the right questions.

"I have gone very close to telling a doctor or two at one stage or another, but it was up to him I think to ask a pertinent question and it didn't happen. I went in to him and I said, 'I have a serious family crisis and I am not dealing with it too well'. He [GP] probed me a little bit on it but he didn't ask the right questions. I expected him to ask me the next question but he didn't. He didn't ask me whether it was a death, whether it was a break up, whether it was 'coming out', whatever it was. Or maybe I should have told him, but he didn't ask the right questions. So it never 'came out'. I felt if he thought it was important enough he would have asked what was the family crisis?" (Gay man)

10.3 All Health Settings

◦ Improve confidentiality and privacy in service settings

"A reception area that has an area of seclusion, just a little area if you were up at the reception desk asking about something, or talking across the desk, getting lab results, a side cubby hole, just something" (Lesbian)

Participants highlighted the need to pay more attention to the provision of private areas (where personal details and discussions cannot be overheard) and to the confidentiality of documents and personal records. They suggested the need to state clearly to people that what is being discussed will be confidential and how this can be assured.

"I think confidentiality is just key, absolutely key. In the area of documentation, I suppose, health care professionals of all grades document a lot, so what would be documented? If I'm telling you a story or telling you about me, how much of that is going to be on my records? I think that is a big issue for [LGB] people. Whereas if I was informed that this is an informal discussion, nothing will be documented unless you want me to, [that also] may help" (Gay man)

◦ Provide, display and disseminate appropriate information, particularly for young LGB people and their families

"I would like them [health care providers] to know a little bit more about the help services for LGB people. It's not that they don't want to know, they just don't know. I'd say they would have no problem doing it but it would be helpful to have the number there to go, 'Okay you're feeling a bit down about your sexuality, here's a number that you can ring'" (Lesbian)

Participants suggested that health care providers take a more proactive role in the provision, display and distribution of information for LGB supports, particularly for young LGB people and their families. This information could be sourced through local LGB support groups or designed in-house in consultation with the LGB community.

"I would expect to see in every GP office an AIDS West, AIDS information, AIDS and STDs helpline, and also something on the North West Lesbian Line. Something offering you know, 'Do you think you might be gay?' Some information, some flier that looks after the mental health side of things as well. Every other mental health support service can be there but that one often isn't. A directory where a person could just have access to flick through, because if you pick up a brochure you know people might be watching [you]" (Lesbian)

"They must accommodate for issues that are there for gay and lesbian people, particularly 'coming out' issues for young people. That information is freely available, and confidentiality can be assured because it's difficult for young gay people. That there is a one-stop shop of maybe one A4 sheet with a list of numbers and names. Maybe leaflets. For parents as well, the possibility they would have gay children and how to deal with that. Take more opportunities to have information out there, so that they don't necessarily have to be going whispering to somebody looking for it" (Gay man)

10.4 Particular Health Settings

◦ *Understand and meet the needs of LGB people in sexual health services*

Participants made a number of suggestions regarding ways of ensuring that sexual health services could more specifically meet the needs of the LGB population. These include:

- Establish a GUM clinic in County Donegal.
- Improve sexual and reproductive health services and information for lesbians.
- Provide more support and counselling – particularly in relation to HIV testing.
- Design and disseminate sexual health information that takes account of LGB people.
- Consider the provision of specialised sexual health services, for example a lesbian sexual health clinic or HIV awareness clinic.

"There should be more information on issues like STDs for lesbians. There is absolutely nothing, there is nowhere that you can find information like that. As a young person myself and I haven't been in many relationships – any. I find it hard to know like where to go, where to ask those questions. Maybe for the GUM [clinic] to advertise that [for] one hour a week there will be a lesbian based here that they will understand your issues, then you can go in and talk to them about any issues that you have, that's a start" (Lesbian)

◦ *Understand and meet the needs of LGB people in mental health services*

"I would wish that they [service providers] could understand the psychology of sexuality, I suppose, and understand the effect particularly of trying to hide the sexuality. It's a mental health issue trying to cover that up and how that warps other areas within life. It's about understanding that and I feel that there's no appreciation of that … I can only speak from my experience as a gay man, how that has affected me down my life. To have them [health care providers] totally dismiss that – to me it was the most important thing – it was very undermining" (Gay man)

Participants suggested that the following issues be addressed by mental health care providers in order to understand and meet the needs of LGB people:

- Cease the practice of pathologising homosexuality.
- Acknowledge how pressures from societal attitudes towards homosexuality and bisexuality can impact on the mental health of LGB people particularly in relation to self-esteem and health-related behaviours (especially at an early age).
- Identify potential lifelines for LGB people (e.g. outside supports/contacts/groups).
- Do not ignore or minimise the importance of sexual orientation to mental health.
- Do not presume that the mental ill-health of an LGB client is necessarily linked to their sexual identity.
- Provide more tailored and LGB-sensitive support and counselling.
- Highlight practices that are 'LGB-friendly'.

◦ Understand and meet the needs of LGB people in GP services

"I suppose it would be nice if there was, if you'd seen something in the post, or there was something up in the surgery to say that if you're gay that there's no problem and that you should admit this to your doctor" (Gay man)

Participants suggested that GPs address the following issues in order to understand and meet the needs of LGB people:

- Understand how pressures from societal attitudes towards homosexuality and bisexuality can impact on LGB health.
- Identify potential lifelines for LGB people (e.g. outside supports, information and contacts).
- Do not ignore sexual orientation – acknowledge and demonstrate an understanding of the issue.
- Provide more tailored and LGB-sensitive support and counselling.
- Provide relevant and tailored information.
- Enhance the visibility of LGB issues within the service (e.g. provide LGB posters, leaflets and other literature in waiting areas).

"Obviously a gay person will feel comfortable if they look up on the wall and they do see something. Or they pick up a leaflet and yes, it is dealing with gay issues or some gay rights sort of thing. Because then it does say yes, well, there is someone here, you know in the [GP] surgery, they are not afraid that gay people do exist and do need treatments as well as anyone else does" (Gay man)

10.5 The LGB Community

◦ Take more responsibility for setting the context of sexual identity issues with the service provider and be open when medically necessary

Some participants identified the need for LGB people to take more responsibility as clients for setting out sexuality issues with the service provider and to be more open about sexual identity, where possible.

"People should take responsibility for their own health, which means informing the practitioner that they have chosen to employ to help them, informing them of all the relevant information. Sometimes relevant information is not always easy to get across if we're having angst about it, but if the patient – I hate that word – is taking responsibility for their health and they've taken the step of actually going to seek some assistance, then they should support themselves and aid the practitioner when it's relevant by giving them that piece of information" (Lesbian)

"As to the physical side of things, I am not saying the patient has to be professional but at least the patient should allow the doctor to do their job. And if he comes around to it, and there's blood involved, I am afraid that you have to tell them [that you're gay]. If there is a problem with you, it's only fair" (Gay man)

"I think we should be asking more of the service providers, 'How comfortable are you? Do you know any LGB people? Have you got any LGB friends?'" (Lesbian)

◦ Collect relevant local information and disseminate accordingly

Some participants suggested the need for the LGB community to collect relevant local information on LGB issues and to provide this to service providers. Some also identified the need to collate a list of LGB-friendly service providers and provide this to the LGB community.

"It seems to be my experience in general that the gay community … sort of looks after the information [on sexual health]. Unless it's done through a setting like a women's conference or lesbian seminars or gay seminars, then those sort of things don't really get talked about" (Lesbian)

"Maybe if the GPs in the area would come forward in some way and let the health board know that you know, 'I would like my name on a leaflet so that people who are gay or lesbian know that I am a gay-friendly doctor and they will not be treated any differently when they come to me" (Lesbian)

11

CONCLUSION

This study uses qualitative methods to record the experience of lesbian, gay and bisexual people in accessing health services in the north west region. Drawing upon the personal testimony of a sample of 43 respondents, obtained through in-depth interviews, it explores their experiences as health service users and their perspectives on the quality of care that they receive. In documenting this lived experience, it illuminates the barriers that can restrict LGB people from accessing the health service on an equal footing with other clients and discusses how those barriers can be addressed. It also considers how good practice can be encouraged at the levels of both the health service organisation and the individual service provider.

This concluding chapter focuses upon the experiences of LGB people and the barriers that prevent them from accessing an equitable health service. It summarises the recommendations of participants concerning how these barriers can be addressed and how good practice can be encouraged. It discusses the two key levels that need to be addressed if access to health care services for LGB people is to be improved: the health system level – its value system or organisational culture and the environment or setting of particular services; and the individual service provider level, including skills, knowledge, attitudes, behaviours and practices at the LGB client–provider interface.

11.1 Barriers to Access

A complexity of behaviours, beliefs and practices operate as barriers to access at many different levels of the health system and have a cumulative effect on the quality of care for many LGB people. Table 11.1 presents a summary of those barriers to accessing services that were reported by the respondents.

Research participants identified the assumption made by health care providers that they were heterosexual as a considerable barrier for them in accessing health-related services. There exists a prevailing assumption across health services in the north west that all service users are heterosexual unless they explicitly declare otherwise. This can have a profound impact on the lives of LGB people who need to access health services when they are sick or require medical advice or attention. It imposes on them an additional burden of having to choose between hiding one of the most fundamental aspects of their lives from the health service professionals whose duty it is to help them – a relationship where trust is paramount – or revealing their LGB sexual identity and leaving themselves open to possible homophobic attitudes and prejudicial behaviour.

Table 11.1: Summary of Barriers to Accessing Health Services for LGB People

Level of influence	Actual or perceived barriers to accessing health services and quality of care for LGB people
Broad societal	• Societal heterosexism and homophobia. • Lack of knowledge or acceptance about LGB people's rights. • Lack of knowledge about LGB people and their health issues. • Keeping it hidden, role of education sector. • Influence of the Catholic Church's perspective on homosexuality on societal values and norms.
Health system (the organisational culture is a microcosm of society)	• Organisational heterosexism and homophobia. • Lack of knowledge or acceptance of the rights of LGB people. • Lack of knowledge about LGB health issues and LGB perspectives. • Invisibility of LGB people in community or health workforce.
Health service setting	• Organisational heterosexism and homophobia. • Invisibility of LGB people in community or health workforce. • Resistance to, or low acceptance of, same-sex partners as next of kin. • Lack of appropriate information available on LGB health and issues.
Individual service provider	• Own attitudes to homosexuality, possible homophobia, religious beliefs. • Lack of knowledge or acceptance about LGB people's rights. • Lack of knowledge/training on LGB health issues and perspectives. • Lack of skills in dealing appropriately with LGB clients and health issues. • Own level of exposure to LGB people within family or friends circle.
LGB client–provider interface	• Tendency to/risk of assumption of heterosexuality. • Inappropriate or homophobic reactions to disclosure. • Asking the wrong questions, missing/not knowing potential lifelines. • Lack of appropriate information/supports available for LGB client. • Minimising sexual identity in overall health and well-being of LGB client. • Not taking a holistic view of LGB person's health, focus on disease or situation and not context of the person's life and social networks.
Individual LGB client	• Level of confidence in being 'out'. • Possible internalised homophobia. • Fear for personal safety. • Expectation or previous experience of a negative reaction to disclosure of sexual identity. • Concerns over trust and confidentiality. • Leaving the region for care. • Delaying or avoiding seeking care at all. • Lack of community supports and social networks.

Although a small proportion of the research participants reported overtly negative comments regarding their LGB sexuality, more subtle forms of homophobia were more commonly experienced. These included inappropriate questioning, changing the subject or ignoring sexuality-related issues and the apparent discomfort of some service providers as observed through their body language. Heterosexism was experienced through questioning that assumed participants were in relationships with opposite-sex partners, a lack of information on LGB health issues and a lack of visibility of LGB people within health service settings. Participants' anxiety levels were raised by experiencing a lack of understanding of their situation as LGB people or by having concerns that they would not be understood. They also had concerns about potential reactions to disclosure of LGB sexuality, either due to earlier negative experiences or because of their awareness that wider societal heterosexism and homophobia might be reflected within health-related services. This dilemma regarding disclosure of their sexual identity immediately puts LGB people at a disadvantage in terms of accessing health services and undermines the principle of delivering and receiving equitable health care services.

Participants experience the stress of dealing with the assumptions that they are part of the socially privileged heterosexual majority, as set out by Eliason (2000), by having to pretend they are of this group or having to disclose that they are not. This concern about experiencing heterosexism and homophobia had a number of negative outcomes for the participants, similar to those documented elsewhere (Dillon and Collins, 2004). These included withholding sensitive and sexuality-related information, avoiding or delaying accessing appropriate services and travelling elsewhere to access services, which could lead to local service providers not having relevant information about clients.

11.2 Recommendations of Respondents

The evidence from the interviews clearly shows that to achieve any improvements in access and quality the first fundamental requirement is that health service providers understand the nature of the lived experience of the LGB person accessing care and how LGB people define the quality of that care. A number of possible changes to the overall service setting and organisational culture, as well as to the behaviour of individual service providers, are then needed to facilitate an improvement in access.

Table 11.2 summarises the recommendations of respondents as to how the barriers that prevent them from accessing an equitable health service can be addressed and how good practice can be encouraged. These suggestions include specific actions for the health system generally, for all health care providers, for particular service settings and for LGB people themselves. Collectively, they represent a roadmap of 'steps in the right direction' to enhance the experience of using health services for LGB clients.

Table 11.2: Summary of Suggestions to Improve Access to Health Services

For the organisation	<ul><li>Emphasise a culture of 'equal rights' rather than 'special treatment'.</li><li>Counter heterosexism and homophobia throughout the organisation.</li><li>Acknowledge that both service users and staff may be LGB and raise the visibility of the group throughout the health service.</li><li>Introduce and influence more training on LGB issues and the social context and on medical issues specific to LGB patients.</li><li>Form partnerships with the LGB community.</li><li>Work proactively with the education sector.</li><li>Address issues of same-sex partners and next of kin in health care settings.</li></ul>
For all service providers	<ul><li>Seek and secure training about LGB issues and perspectives and about specific medical issues for LGB people.</li><li>Do not assume clients are heterosexual; be more accepting of difference.</li><li>If an LGB client decides to disclose her/his sexual identity, react appropriately.</li><li>Be sensitive to what stage an LGB client is at in the process of 'coming out'.</li></ul>
For all service settings	<ul><li>Improve confidentiality and privacy.</li><li>Disseminate appropriate information, particularly for young LGB people.</li></ul>
For particular services	<ul><li>Understand and meet the needs of LGB people in sexual health services.</li><li>Understand and meet the needs of LGB people in mental health services.</li><li>Understand and meet the needs of LGB people in GP services.</li></ul>
For LGB people	<ul><li>Take more responsibility for setting the context with the service provider.</li><li>Collect relevant local information and supply it to service providers.</li></ul>

11.3 Actions Required by the Health System

This study has charted new territory by conducting primary qualitative research into the experience of a hitherto invisible group – a predominantly rural LGB community – whose needs have never before been explicitly acknowledged or wholly met by the public health service. Arising from this study, the most pressing change at the structural level is for the HSE to play a leadership role in countering heterosexism and homophobia in the organisation. This research is a small but significant first step in that process of engagement with LGB people to identify their service needs. The HSE should build upon it by placing LGB equality issues at the centre of service planning and policy development and by forming further partnerships with LGB organisations to comprehensively challenge heterosexism within the health system.

A key message emerging from the study is that the HSE needs to address the invisibility of LGB people within the context both of service delivery and of the HSE workforce. It can do this by explicitly identifying and acknowledging the health care needs of LGB service users/patients in informational, promotional and educational documentation and resource materials that are available in core health care settings such as hospitals and primary care centres. Participants in the research were clear that one key dimension of providing an appropriate service to LGB people is that procedures must be put in place by the HSE that acknowledge same-sex partners as next of kin in health care settings.

Another crucial change at the system level would be for the HSE to provide sensitivity and awareness training to improve the knowledge and skills of service providers in understanding and dealing with LGB people and their health care needs. There is a consensus amongst the research respondents that primary care, sexual health and mental health professionals in particular should have specialist training around LGB health issues. Furthermore, service providers, in particular GPs, need to be aware of the concerns of lesbians regarding disclosure of sexual identity, confidentiality and sensitive practice in relation to sexual/gynaecological health, to ensure that as a group they are not discouraged from accessing these essential medical services. Changes such as these would represent a major strategic shift towards making the environment more inclusive of LGB people both in the organisation of the health system and in the culture of the settings where health care is delivered.

11.4 Actions Required by Individual Health Care Providers

The recommendations of this research do not just apply to the system level of the health service organisation. If the needs of LGB people are to be properly addressed it requires individual health care providers to evaluate their practice and to change their behaviour as appropriate. Every individual with a responsibility to deliver a service within the health system at any level, from the most senior to the most junior, needs to understand this process, to make constant efforts to counter heterosexism and homophobia and to be more understanding of the needs of LGB people. This means that all health care providers should be open to the possibility that any client may be lesbian, gay or bisexual rather than assuming that all clients are heterosexual. It requires that they be sensitive to the vulnerability LGB people may feel in disclosing their sexual identity and respond appropriately with reassurance and acceptance.

The research suggests that confidentiality between practitioner and service user/patient is an issue that is particularly salient for LGB people who need to be fully convinced that they can trust their health professionals with sensitive or personal information. Furthermore, while it is the responsibility of the HSE to ensure that evidence-based information on LGB health issues is available, there is also an onus on individual service providers to ensure that this literature is disseminated in all health service facilities.

In the research, emotional and mental health was the main health issue identified by participants – only four participants did not mention emotional or mental health matters in the course of the interviews. There is a responsibility on service providers to understand the particular experiences of LGB people as members of a marginalised group that may be subject to additional mental health pressures due to their acquaintance with heterosexism and homophobia. On a practical level, this requires that mental health professionals, when treating people who may be distressed or suicidal, are sensitive to the possibility that their clients may be experiencing difficulties with sexuality issues, and respond supportively.

11.5 Further Research

This research identified concerns that the social stigmatisation of LGB sexual orientation may contribute to increased risk of suicide and self-harm. Yet LGB sexuality is largely absent from suicide prevention policies in Ireland and the issue of LGB sexual identity as a causal factor has not to date been addressed in national research on suicide in Ireland. This lack of information suggests that primary research is necessary to identify the significance of LGB sexual orientation as a factor in suicide or self-harm in Ireland. In the meantime, those engaged in suicide prevention work need to address LGB sexual identity within suicide prevention policies and practices.

This is the first official research conducted on the health care needs of the LGB community in the north west. It presents the HSE and individual service providers with a clear agenda for change that is informed by the actual voices of local LGB people and it calls for appropriate services that recognise their specific health care needs as a group. However, if the necessary changes are to be successfully integrated into the planning and delivery of health services, further research will be required to examine the views of health service professionals on how they feel they are currently serving their LGB clients and how best they can be supported to provide a better, more equitable service in the future.

APPENDIX

Table A1: GP-Related Health Issues Considered Most Important for LGB Clients

	Lesbians	Gay men	Total
Sexual health	11	16	27
Mental health	10	9	19
Next of kin	6	0	6
Maternity/parenting	6	0	6
Blood-testing	0	3	3
Transgender issues	0	1	1

Table A2: Hospitalisation Issues for LGB Clients

	Lesbians	Gay men	Total
Next of kin/partnership isues	11	5	16
Confidentiality concerns	2	5	7
Fear of negative reaction to disclosure	6	1	7
Assumption of heterosexuality by hospital staff	3	2	5

Table A3: Frequency of Interviewees' References to Mental Health

	Lesbians (n=24)	Gay men (n=19)
Interviewees that attended mental health services (including GPs)	14	12
Additional interviewees that referred to mental health as an issue for LGB health care	7	6
Interviews where mental health issues arose	21	18

Table A4: Degree of Disclosure of LGB Sexual Identity

		Lesbians	Gay men	Total
Family	All	16	9	25
	Some	7	5	12
	None	1	5	6
	Total	24	19	43
Friends	All	23	12	35
	Some	1	7	8
	None	0	0	0
	Total	24	19	43
Work/college	All	12	8	20
	Some	6	4	10
	None	6	5	11
	Total	24	17	41

Table A5: Rate of Disclosure of LGB Sexual Identity to Health Services

	Lesbians	Gay men	Total
All health services	4	5	9
Some health services	12	10	22
No health services	8	4	12
Total	24	19	43

Table A6: Rate of Disclosure of LGB Sexual Identity to Mental Health Professionals (excluding GPs)

	No. occasions sexuality disclosed	No. occasions sexuality not disclosed	Total
NWHB psychiatrists	10	2	12
Other HSE mental health practitioners	17	5	22
Private mental health practitioners	14	0	14
Total	41	7	48

Table A7: Health Issues Associated with Disclosure of LGB Sexual Identity to GP Services

	Lesbians (n=12)	Gay men (n=11)	Total (n=23)
Mental health	6	7	13
Sexual health	6	4	10
Gynaecological/obstetrical health	3	0	3
Medical history/GP query	2	1	3
Blood tests	0	2	2
Other issues related to sexuality	2	0	2
Total incidents of disclosure	19	14	33

Table A8: Rate of Attendance for Mental Health Support during Study Period

	Lesbians (n=24)	Gay men (n=19)	Total (n=43)
GP only	1	3	4
Both GP and other mental health professionals	6	4	10
Mental health professionals only	7	5	12
Total	14	12	26

Table A9: Main Reasons Cited for Attending Mental Health Professionals (excluding GPs)

	Lesbians	Gay men	Total
Depression/suicidal feelings associated with LGB sexual identity	4	4	8
Discomfort with LGB sexual identity	4	2	6
History of child sexual abuse	5	1	6
Living 'in the closet'/ homophobia of family	3	1	4
Difficult marriage relationships	2	0	2
Other	4	4	8

REFERENCES

Adamson, JA and Donovan, JL (2002) 'Qualitative research in black and white: the insider/outsider debate', *Qualitative Health Research,* 12(6): 816–825

Albarran, JW and Salmon, D (2000) 'Lesbian, gay and bisexual experiences within critical care nursing, 1988–1998: a survey of the literature', *International Journal of Nursing Studies,* 37: 445–455

American Psychological Association (2000) 'Guidelines for psychotherapy with lesbian, gay and bisexual clients', *American Psychologist,* 55(12): 1440–1451

APA, American Psychiatric Association (2000) 'Position statement on therapies focused on attempts to change sexual orientation (reparative or conversion therapies)', *American Journal of Psychiatry,* 157(10): 1719–1721

Barron, M and Collins, E (2005) 'Responding to the needs of vulnerable lesbian, gay, bisexual and transgendered youth', paper presented at the Irish Association of Suicidology Fifth Annual Conference, Dublin, December

Bartlett, A, Michael, K and Phillips, P (2001) 'Straight talking: an investigation of the attitudes and practice of psychoanalysts and psychotherapists in relation to gays and lesbians', *British Journal of Psychiatry,* 179: 545–549

Becknell, JM (1994) 'Gays in the EMS: strengthening the EMS team', *Journal of Emergency Medicine,* 19(8): 94–100

BeLonG To (2005) 'LGBT youth and suicide', submission to the National Strategy for Action on Suicide Prevention, Dublin: BeLonG To

Berkman, C and Zinberg, G (1997) 'Homophobia and heterosexism in social workers', *Social Work,* 42(4): 319–332

Boehmer, U (2002) 'Twenty years of public health research: inclusion of lesbian, gay, bisexual and transgender populations', *American Journal of Public Health,* 92(7): 1125–1130

Bradford, J, Ryan, C and Rothblum, ED (1994) 'National Lesbian Health Care Survey: implications for mental health care', *Journal of Consulting and Clinical Psychology,* 62: 228–242

Bradford, J, Ryan, C, Honed, J and Rothblum, E (2001) 'Expanding the research infrastructure for lesbian health', *American Journal of Public Health,* 91(7): 1029–1032

Braveman, PA (2003) 'Monitoring equity in health and healthcare: a conceptual framework', *Journal of Health, Population and Nutrition,* 3: 181–192

Brotman, S, Ryan, NB, Jalbert, Y and Rowe, B (2002) 'The impact of coming out on health and health care access: the experiences of gay, lesbian, bisexual and two spirit people', *Journal of Health and Social Policy,* 15(1): 1–29

Cain, R (1991) 'Disclosure and secrecy among gay men in the United States and Canada: a shift in views', J*ournal of the History of Sexuality,* 2(1): 25–45

Chaimowitz, GA (1991) 'Homophobia among psychiatric residents, family practice residents and psychiatric faculty', *Canadian Journal of Psychiatry,* 36(3): 206–209

Carolan, F and Redmond, S (2003) *ShOut: Research into the Needs of Young People in Northern Ireland who Identify as Lesbian, Gay, Bisexual and/or Transgender,* Belfast: YouthNet

Carr, SV (1999) 'A community-based lesbian health service: clinically justified or just politically correct?', *British Journal of Family Planning,* 25(3): 93–95

CIOMS, Council for International Organisations of Medical Sciences (1993) *International Ethical Guidelines for Biomedical Research Involving Human Subjects,* Geneva: CIOMS

Combat Poverty Agency and Equality Authority (2003) *Poverty and Inequality: Applying an Equality Dimension to Poverty Proofing,* Dublin: Combat Poverty Agency/Equality Authority

Cooper, D (1994) *Sexing the City: Lesbian and Gay Politics within the Activist State,* London: Rivers Oram Press

Denenberg, R. (1995) 'Report on lesbian health', *Women's Health International,* 5(2), 81–91

Diamant, AL and Wold, C (2003) 'Sexual orientation and variation in physical and mental health status among women', *Journal of Women's Health,* 12(1): 41–49

Diamant, AL, Schuster, MA and Lever, J (2000a) 'Receipt of preventive health care services by lesbians', *American Journal of Preventive Medicine,* 19(3): 141–148

Diamant, AL, Wold, C, Spritzer, K and Geldberg, L (2000b) 'Health behaviours, health status and access to and use of health care: a population-based study of lesbian, bisexual and heterosexual women', *Archives of Family Medicine,* 9(10): 1043–1051

Dibble, SL, Roberts, SA, Robertson, PA and Paul, SM (2002) 'Risk factors for ovarian cancer: lesbian and heterosexual women', *Oncology Nursing Forum,* 29(1): E1–7

Dillon, A (1999) 'Lesbian health in Ireland', policy document, Dublin: Lesbian Education and Awareness

Dillon, B and Collins, E (2004) *Mental Health, Lesbians and Gay Men: Developing Strategies to Counter the Impact of Social Exclusion and Stigmatization,* Dublin: Gay HIV Strategies and the Northern Area Health Board

DOHC, Department of Health and Children (1997) *A Plan for Women's Health,* Dublin: Stationery Office

DOHC, Department of Health and Children (2000) *The National Health Promotion Strategy 2000–2005,* Dublin: Stationery Office

DOHC, Department of Health and Children (2001) *Get Connected – Developing an Adolescent Friendly Health Service,* Dublin: DOHC

DOHC, Department of Health and Children (2002) 'Circular: Equality Authority Report: "Implementing Equality for Lesbians, Gays and Bisexuals"', Dublin: DOHC

DOHC, Department of Health and Children (2006) *A Vision for Change, Report of the Expert Group on Mental Health Policy,* Dublin: DOHC

Eliason, MJ (2000) 'Substance abuse counsellors' attitudes regarding lesbian, gay, bisexual and transgendered clients', *Journal of Substance Abuse,* 12(4): 311–328

Equality Authority (2002) *Implementing Equality for Lesbians, Gay and Bisexuals,* Dublin: Equality Authority

Equality Authority, HSE and DOHC (2005) *Equal Status Acts 2000 to 2004 and the Provision of Health Services,* Dublin: Equality Authority

Eth, S (1992) 'Ethical challenges in the treatment of traumatised refugees', *Journal of Traumatic Stress,* 5(1): 103–110

Family Planning Association, UK (2002) *Policy on Human Sexuality,* London: Family Planning Association

Fitzpatrick, R, Dawson, J, Boulton, M, McLean, J, Hart, G and Brookes, M (1994) 'Perceptions of general practice among homosexual men', *British Journal of General Practice,* 44 (379): 80–82

Franke, R and Leary, MR (1991) 'Disclosure of sexual orientation by lesbians and gay men: a comparison of private and public processes', *Journal of Social and Clinical Psychology,* 10: 262–269

Gay HIV Strategies and Nexus Research Cooperative (2000) *Education: Lesbian and Gay Students: Developing Equal Opportunities,* http://www.glen.ie/public/pdfs/Education%20Report% 202000.pdf

Gay HIV Strategies, Nexus Research and Waterford Area Partnership (1999) *Local Development: Lesbians and Gay Men: The Report of a Strategy Development and Capacity-Building Project with the Waterford Gay and Lesbian Community,* http://www.glen.ie/public/pdfs/Waterford%20Final%20Report %201999.pdf

Ginsburg, KR, Winn, RJ, Rudy, BJ, Crawford, J, Zhao, H and Schwarz, DF (2002) 'How to reach sexual minority youth in the health care setting: the teens offer guidance', *Society for Adolescent Medicine,* 31: 407–416

GLEN and Nexus Research Cooperative (1995) *Poverty, Lesbians and Gay Men: The Economic and Social Effects of Discrimination,* Dublin: Combat Poverty Agency

Greco, JA and Glusman, J (1998) 'Providing effective care for gay and lesbian patients', *Patient Care,* 32(12): 159–170

Hall, JM (1999) 'Marginalization revisited: critical, postmodern, and liberation perspectives', *Advances in Nursing Science,* 2(2): 88–102

Harrison, AE and Silenzio, VMB (1996) 'Comprehensive care of lesbian and gay patients and families', *Primary Care: Models of Ambulatory Care,* 23(1): 231–238

Herek, GM (1994) 'Assessing heterosexuals' attitudes towards lesbians and gay men: a review of empirical research with the ATGL scale', in Greene, B and Herek, GM (eds) *Lesbian and Gay Psychology,* vol. 1, Thousand Oaks, CA: Sage: 206–228

Herek, GM and Berrill, KT (1992) *Hate Crimes: Confronting Violence against Lesbians and Gay Men,* London: Sage

Herek, GM, Cogan, JC, Gillis, JR and Glunt, EK (1998) 'Correlates of internalized homophobia in a community sample of lesbians and gay men', *Journal of the Gay and Lesbian Medical Association,* 2(1): 17–25

Hickson, F, Weatherburn, P, Reid, D and Stephens, M (2003) *Out and About: Findings from the United Kingdom's Gay Men's Sex Survey 2002,* original research report, London: Sigma Research, University of Portsmouth with The Terence Higgins Trust, Healthy Gay Scotland, and Community HIV and Aids Prevention Strategy

Hitchcock, JM and Wilson, HS (1992) 'Personal risking: Lesbian disclosure of sexual orientation to professional health care providers', *Nursing Research,* 41(3): 178–183

Holyoake, D (1999) 'Favourite patients: exploring labeling in patient culture', *Nursing Standard,* 13(16): 44–47

HSE and DOHC (2005) *Reach Out: National Strategy for Action on Suicide Prevention 2005–2014,* Dublin: Health Service Executive

Huebner, DM, Davis, MC, Nemeroff, CJ and Aiken, LS (2002) 'The impact of internalized homophobia on HIV preventive interventions', *American Journal of Community Psychology,* 30(3): 327–348

Hughes, D (2004) 'Disclosure of sexual preferences and lesbian, gay and bisexual practitioners', *British Medical Journal,* 328: 1211–1212

Jarman, N and Tennant, A (2003) *An Acceptable Prejudice? Homophobic Violence and Harassment in Northern Ireland,* Belfast: Institute for Conflict Research

Johnson, M and Webb, C (1995) 'Rediscovering unpopular patients: the concept of social judgement', *Journal of Advanced Nursing Studies,* 21: 466–475

Klitzman, RL and Greenberg, JD (2002) 'Patterns of communication between gay and lesbian patients and their health care providers', *Journal of Homosexuality,* 42(4): 65–75

L.Inc (2006) *L.Inc Lesbian Health Research: A Study of the General Health of the Lesbian Community in Cork,* Cork: L.Inc.

Mathews, WMC, Booth, MV, Turner, JD and Kessler, L (1986) 'Physicians' attitudes towards homosexuality – survey of a California county-medical society', *Western Journal of Medicine,* 144: 106–110

Mathieson, CM, Bailey, N and Gurevich, M (2002) 'Health care services for lesbian and bisexual women: some Canadian data', *Health Care for Women International,* 23: 185–190

McManus, S (2003) *Sexual Orientation Research Phase 1: A Review of Methodological Approaches,* Edinburgh: National Centre for Social Research/Scottish Executive Social Research

Mee, J and Ronayne, K (2000) *Partnership Rights for Same-Sex Couples,* Dublin: Equality Authority

Miller, B (2003) 'Fighting sexual prejudice. Report on the first national survey into the health needs of lesbian, gay, bisexual and transgender people (Scotland)', *Health Development Today,* June/July

Morris, JF and Rothblum, ED (1999) 'Who fills out a lesbian questionnaire? The interrelationship of sexual orientation, years out, disclosure of sexual orientation and sexual experiences with women, particularly in the lesbian community', *Psychology of Women Quarterly,* 33: 537–557

Morrisey, M (1996) 'Gay, lesbian and bisexual adolescents providing esteem-enhancing care to a battered population', *The Nurse Practitioner,* 22(2): 94–99

Mullineaux, DG and French, SA (1996) 'Speaking out. Lesbian couples and cancer', *Innovations in Breast Cancer Care,* 1(4): 86–90

Ndofor-Tah, C, Hickson, F, Weatherburn, P, Amamoo, NA, Majekodunmi, Y, Reid, D, Robinson, F, Sanyu-Sseruma, W and Zulu, A (2000) *Capital Assets,* London: Sigma Research

NESF, National Economic and Social Forum (2003) *Equality Policies for Lesbian, Gay and Bisexual People: Implementation Issues,* Forum Report No. 27, Dublin: National Economic and Social Forum

Norman, J, Galvin, M and McNamara, G (2006) *Straight Talk: An Investigation of Attitudes and Experiences of Homophobic Bullying in Second-Level Schools,* Dublin: Dublin City University

Nuffield Council on Bioethics (2002) *Genetics and Human Behaviour: The Ethical Context,* London: Nuffield Council on Bioethics

O'Carroll, I (1999) *A Queer Quandary: The Challenges of Including Sexual Difference within the Relationships and Sexuality Education Programme,* Dublin: Lesbian Education and Awareness

O'Carroll, I and Collins, E (1995) *Lesbians and Gay Visions of Ireland,* London: Cassells

Palmer, H (1996) 'Nursing care of gay men with HIV-related malignancy', *Journal of Cancer Care,* 5(4): 163–167

Ponticelli, CM (ed.) (1998) *Gateways to Improving Lesbian Health and Health Care: Opening Doors,* Binghampton, NY: The Harrington Press

Pringle, A (2003) *Beyond Barriers. Scottish Survey into the Health Needs of Lesbian, Gay, Bisexual and Transgender People,* Glasgow: LGBT Health Project, Stonewall Scotland

Quiery, M (2002) *A Mighty Silence: A Report on the Needs of Lesbians and Bisexual Women in Northern Ireland,* Belfast: Lesbian Advocacy Services Initiative (LASI)

Rankow, EJ (1995) 'Breast and cervical cancer among lesbians', *Women's Health Issues,* 5(3): 123–129

Remafedi, G, French, S and Story, M (1998) 'The relationship between suicide risk and sexual orientation: results of a population-based study', *American Journal of Public Health,* 88(1): 57–60

Riordan, DC (2004) 'Interaction strategies of lesbian, gay and bisexual healthcare practitioners in the clinical examination of patients: qualitative study', *British Medical Journal online,* doi:10:1136/bmj.38071.774525.EB (published 27 April)

Risdon, C, Cook, D and Williams, D (2000) 'Gay and lesbian physicians in training: a qualitative study', *Canadian Medical Association Journal,* 162(3): 331

Rose, K (1998) 'Parallel universes: gay and lesbian issues and local development', in Fahy, K (ed.) *Local Development in Ireland – Policy Implications for the Future,* Galway: Community Workers Co-operative: 134–149

Rose, L (1994) 'Homophobia among doctors', *British Medical Journal,* 308: 586–587

Rose, P (1993) 'Out in the open', *Nursing Times,* 89(30): 50–52

Rose, P and Platzer, H (1993) 'Confronting prejudice', *Nursing Times,* 89(31): 52–54

Saddul, R (1996) 'Coming out: an overlooked concept', *Clinical Nurse Specialist,* 10(1): 2–5

Sarma, K (2007) *Drug Use Amongst Lesbian, Gay, Bisexual & Transgender Young Adults in Ireland,* Dublin: BeLonG To

Schneider, JS and Levin, S (1999) 'Uneasy partners: the lesbian and gay health care community and the AMA (American Medical Association)', *Journal of the American Medical Association,* 282(13): 1287–1288

Smith, EM, Johnson, SR and Guenther, SM (1985) 'Health care attitudes and experiences during gynecologic care among lesbians and bisexuals', *American Journal of Public Health,* 75(9): 1085–1087

Smith, GB (1992) 'Nursing care challenges: homosexual psychiatric patients', *Journal of Psychosocial Nursing,* 30(12): 50–51

Snape, D, Katarina, T and Chetwynd, M (1995) *Discrimination Against Gay Men and Lesbians: A Study of the Nature and Extent of Discrimination Against Homosexual Men and Women in Britain Today,* London: SCPR

Stevens, PE (1995) 'Structural and interpersonal impact of heterosexual assumptions on lesbian health care clients', *Nursing Research,* 44(1): 25–37

Stevens, PE (1998) 'The experiences of lesbians of colour in health care encounters: narrative insights for improving access and quality', in Ponticelli, CM (ed.) *Gateways to Improving Lesbian Health and Health Care: Opening Doors,* Binghampton, NY: The Haworth Press: 77–94

Stewart, M (1999) 'Lesbian parents talk about their birth experiences', *British Journal of Midwifery,* 7(2): 96–101

Taillon, R (1999) *Needs Analysis: Lesbians and Bisexual Women in the Dublin Area,* Dublin: Nexus Research Co-operative

Trotter, J (1999) 'Lesbian and gay issues in work with young people: are schools "out" this summer?', *British Journal of Social Work,* 29: 995–961

Turner, G and Mallet, L (1998) 'A second survey of the health needs of gay and lesbian issues in child and adolescent psychiatry training as reported by training directors', *Journal of the American Academy of Child and Adolescent Psychiatry,* 36(6): 764–768

US Committee on Human Sexuality (2000) *Homosexuality and the Mental Health Professions: The Impact of Bias,* Hillsdale, NJ: Analytic Press

Van Voorhis, R and Wagner, M (2002) 'Among the missing: content on lesbian and gay people in social work journals', *Social Work,* 47(4): 345–354

Walpin, L (1997) 'Combating heterosexism: implications for nursing', *Clinical Nurse Specialist,* 11(3): 126–132

Wardlaw, C (1994) *One in Every Family: Myths about Lesbians and Gay Men,* Dublin: Basement Press

Wells, A (1997) 'Homophobia and nursing', *Nursing Standard,* 12(6): 41–42

White, J and Martinez, CM (eds) (1997) *The Lesbian Health Book—Caring for Ourselves,* Seattle: Seal Press

Wilkinson, R and Marmot, M (2003) *Social Determinants of Health: The Solid Facts* (2nd edn), Copenhagen: WHO Regional Office for Europe

Wilton, T (1996) 'Caring for the lesbian client: homophobia and midwifery', *British Journal of Midwifery,* 4(3): 126–131

Wilton, T (1999) 'Towards an understanding of the cultural roots of homophobia in order to provide a better midwifery service for lesbian clients', *Midwifery,* 15(3): 165–176

Women's Health Council (2003) 'Women, disadvantage and health: a position paper of The Women's Health Council', Dublin: Women's Health Council

Working Group on Domestic Partnership (2006) *Options Paper,* Dublin: Department of Justice, Equality and Law Reform

World Medical Association (2004) *Declaration of Helsinki: Ethical Principles for Medical Research Involving Human Subjects,* http://www.wma.net/e/policy/b3.htm

Yom, SS (1999) 'Gay men and lesbians in medicine: has discrimination left the room?', *Journal of the American Medical Association,* 282(13): 1286